MW00851272

5-INGREDIENT RENAL DIET COOKBOOK

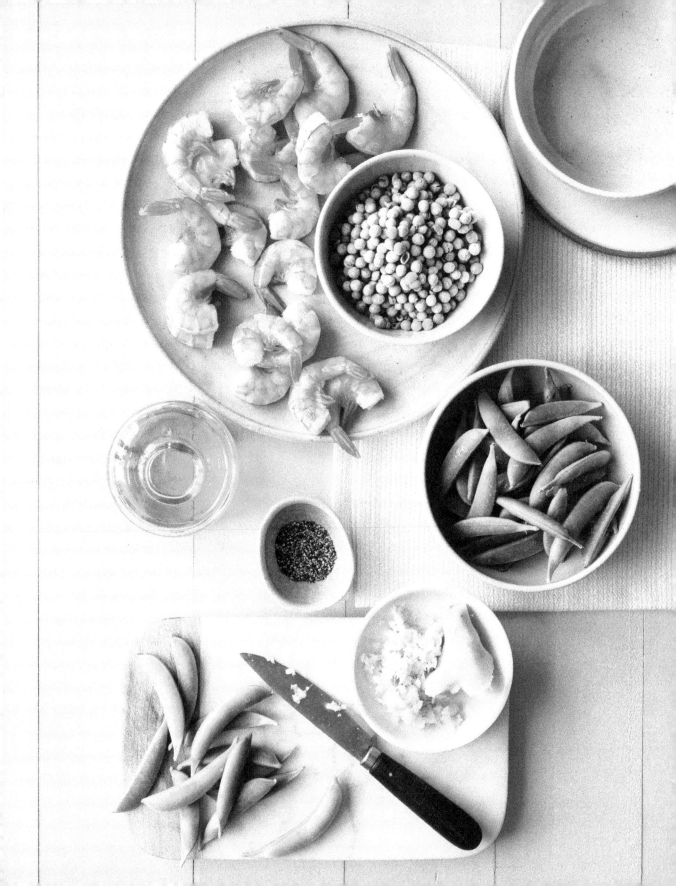

5-Ingredient
RENAL
DIET
COOKBOOK

Quick and Easy Recipes for
Every Stage of Kidney Disease

Aisling Whelan, MS, RDN, CDN

Photography by Nadine Greeff

**ROCKRIDGE
PRESS**

Copyright © 2020 by Rockridge Press, Emeryville, California

No part of this publication may be reproduced, stored in a retrieval system, or transmitted in any form or by any means, electronic, mechanical, photocopying, recording, scanning, or otherwise, except as permitted under Sections 107 or 108 of the 1976 United States Copyright Act, without the prior written permission of the Publisher. Requests to the Publisher for permission should be addressed to the Permissions Department, Rockridge Press, 6005 Shellmound Street, Suite 175, Emeryville, CA 94608.

Limit of Liability/Disclaimer of Warranty: The Publisher and the author make no representations or warranties with respect to the accuracy or completeness of the contents of this work and specifically disclaim all warranties, including without limitation warranties of fitness for a particular purpose. No warranty may be created or extended by sales or promotional materials. The advice and strategies contained herein may not be suitable for every situation. This work is sold with the understanding that the Publisher is not engaged in rendering medical, legal, or other professional advice or services. If professional assistance is required, the services of a competent professional person should be sought. Neither the Publisher nor the author shall be liable for damages arising herefrom. The fact that an individual, organization, or website is referred to in this work as a citation and/or potential source of further information does not mean that the author or the Publisher endorses the information the individual, organization, or website may provide or recommendations they/it may make. Further, readers should be aware that websites listed in this work may have changed or disappeared between when this work was written and when it is read.

For general information on our other products and services or to obtain technical support, please contact our Customer Care Department within the United States at (866) 744-2665, or outside the United States at (510) 253-0500.

Rockridge Press publishes its books in a variety of electronic and print formats. Some content that appears in print may not be available in electronic books, and vice versa.

TRADEMARKS: Rockridge Press and the Rockridge Press logo are trademarks or registered trademarks of Callisto Media Inc. and/or its affiliates, in the United States and other countries, and may not be used without written permission. All other trademarks are the property of their respective owners. Rockridge Press is not associated with any product or vendor mentioned in this book.

Interior and Cover Designer: Michael Cook

Art Producer: Sue Bischofberger

Editor: Britt Bogan

Production Editor: Jenna Dutton

Photography © 2020 Nadine Greeff

Author photo courtesy of Andee Maher

Cover: Pineapple-Soy Salmon Stir-Fry

ISBN: Print 978-1-64611-519-8 | eBook 978-1-64611-520-4

R0

To JJ, my beautiful baby boy.

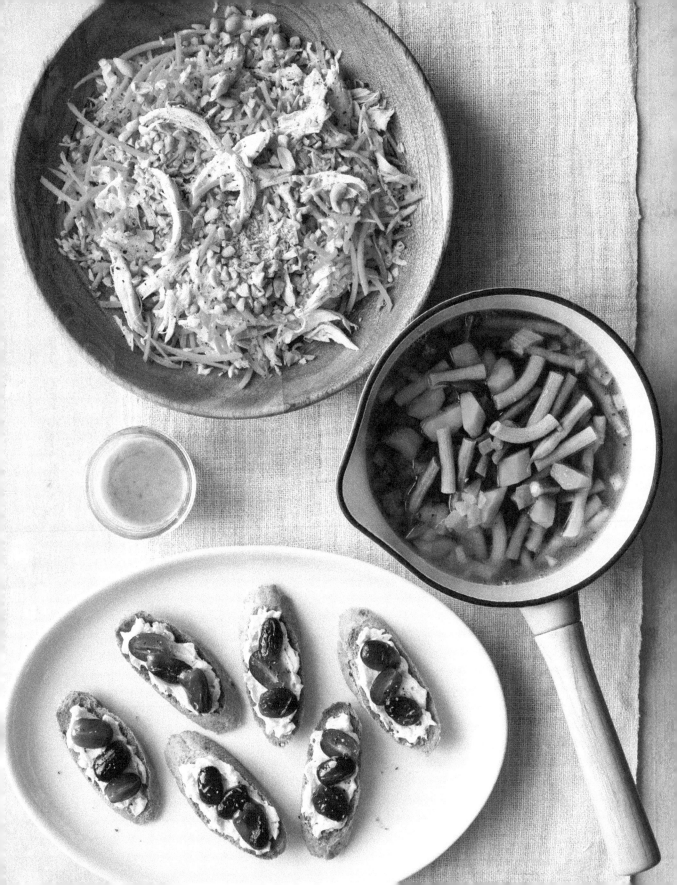

CONTENTS

Introduction

If you or someone close to you has been diagnosed with chronic kidney disease (CKD) and are struggling with what to eat, rest assured. You've come to the right place! Nutrition is a powerful weapon in the fight against CKD, and this book has everything you need to harness its power. As a renal dietitian, I have witnessed many patients successfully slow down or even halt the progression of their CKD with dietary changes. For those on dialysis, the right balance of nutrition can help you feel better, boost your quality of life, and decrease your chances of experiencing future complications. You might worry that in order to achieve success, you'll need to part ways with your favorite foods and commit to a strict and joyless diet forever. I promise that it doesn't have to be this way! You can improve your health and quality of life by eating foods that are both nourishing *and* delicious.

The traditional renal diet focuses mainly on eliminating certain foods to keep lab results such as potassium and phosphorus in the normal range. While this is often important, it's also important that non-dialysis CKD patients adhere to a diet that slows down the rate of kidney function decline. In my experience, most patients are unaware of the profound impact that adding foods *into* their diet can have on their health and disease state. In addition, due to outdated information on the Internet or advice from well-meaning but ill-informed practitioners, many patients unnecessarily restrict certain foods from their diet and feel significantly deprived of options.

Nutritional counseling provided by a renal expert can help clear up confusion around the renal diet in a couple of sessions. Instead of feeling frustrated and anxious, patients begin to feel confident and motivated in their ability to make the changes necessary for their health. A recent client of mine cried tears of relief at our first appointment because she finally felt confident in her ability to take control of her condition through dietary means. After a few months of following my recommendations, she happily reported improvements in several of her lab values. Instead of being told by her doctor that her kidney function had declined further, she was delighted to hear that her kidney function had stabilized! Her doctor advised her to keep doing what she was doing because "it was clearly working."

A CKD diagnosis can lead to many unwelcome changes in your life, such as frequent doctor visits, needing to take several new medications, or the knowledge that your diet needs to be adjusted. With all of this on your plate, it's no wonder that meal preparation can suddenly become a daunting task. This cookbook's purpose is to share with you the wisdom I've gathered from my experience working with patients across the full spectrum of CKD. I'll be keeping the recipes simple, as long lists of ingredients can overwhelm even the most ambitious of cooks. The book sticks to recipes that require five ingredients or less, and many will require only one pot or pan. In addition to recipes, you'll get the information you need to make informed decisions when planning your daily meals. This information is derived from the latest evidenced-based nutrition guidelines for CKD and the clinical experience of expert renal dietitians, such as myself. The kitchen is your lab and now you have the power and knowledge to make the best medicine—food. The first recipe you choose is the first step in the right direction.

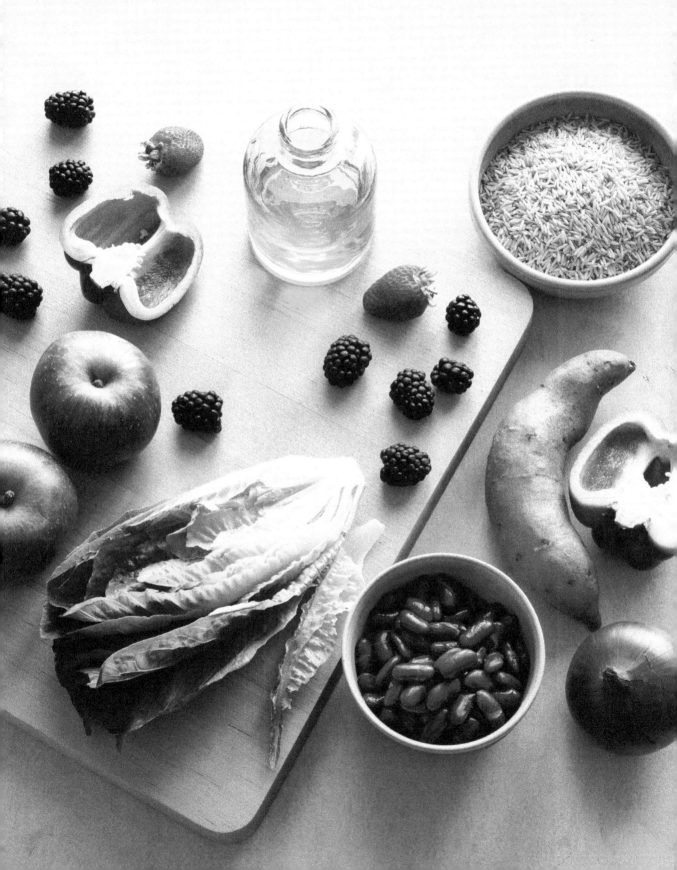

CHAPTER 1

Easy Renal Diet Cooking

THIS chapter outlines the basics of chronic kidney disease (CKD), and explains how the renal diet supports kidney function. This chapter will discuss the foods that need to be limited as well as the foods that should be included in a healthy renal diet. It may get a little "sciencey" at times, but bear with me. It's important that you understand the impact diet has on CKD so that you can make informed food choices and be empowered with the knowledge to improve your health.

WHAT IS CHRONIC KIDNEY DISEASE?

In CKD, the kidneys gradually lose their functional abilities. This loss of function usually happens over months or years, and it frequently occurs without any symptoms in the early stages. Since CKD tends not to be discovered until it has already progressed, it has been referred to as a "silent disease."

Your doctor evaluates your kidney function by performing several tests. A urine analysis looks for abnormalities in the urine such as blood or protein. Blood or protein in the urine can be indicative of renal damage. A test to determine your glomerular filtration rate (GFR) is another common kidney function test. GFR is the measure of how much blood filters through your kidneys each minute. Your GFR is calculated by looking at your blood creatinine level, race, age, and gender. Generally, the lower your GFR, the more advanced the kidney disease.

What Causes CKD?

Though there are many causes of CKD, hypertension and diabetes are two of the most common conditions that contribute to the diagnosis. Hypertension is a disease characterized by excessive pressure in the blood, and diabetes is a disease characterized by excessive sugar. The nephrons are the filtering units of the kidneys, and each kidney contains approximately 1 million of them. The nephrons are very sensitive to the effects of excessive pressure and excessive sugar, and over time these conditions can damage the kidneys' nephrons, reducing their ability to perform their important job of filtering the blood.

The Five Stages of CKD

CKD is classified by five stages. Markers of kidney damage, such as blood or protein in the urine, combined with your GFR level helps your doctor determine what stage of CKD you are in. People in stage 1 and 2 CKD typically do not know they have the disease. That's because in the beginning of CKD, the kidneys do a good job at compensating for the mild damage, and your body continues to function normally without any symptoms presenting. As kidney function declines further, abnormalities may start to show up in your lab work, urine analysis, or blood pressure. When GFR drops below a level of 15 mL/minute (normal is above 60 mL/minute), a person is considered to be in stage 5 CKD, also known as end-stage renal disease. When end-stage renal disease is diagnosed, kidney function has declined to the point where dialysis is required or a kidney transplant is necessary to survive.

How the Renal Diet Supports Kidney Function

Traditionally, the renal diet was all about cutting things out and keeping certain things "low." People were given a one-size-fits-all diet that oftentimes failed to take into consideration a person's stage of CKD or their particular lab values. A more modern approach to the renal diet takes the stance that each person with CKD deserves an individually tailored diet plan. While it's usually true that certain nutrients, such as protein, will need to be kept low if your goal is to delay CKD progression, your individual lab trends will dictate whether other nutrients, such as potassium, need to be as strictly limited.

The traditional renal diet's biggest downfall is that it neglected to focus on the dietary pattern that could most successfully combat some of the key drivers of CKD: chronic inflammation and acid buildup (*acidosis*). These drivers hasten the progression of CKD over time. Diet can play a powerful role in treating CKD because many foods have natural anti-inflammatory and acid-neutralizing properties. When it comes to supporting kidney function, wholesome plant foods are essential to include and should be the foundation of your diet. Practically speaking, this category includes minimally processed foods of plant origin, such as fruits, vegetables, nuts, whole grains, legumes, and olive oil.

In addition to their many anti-inflammatory compounds, many wholesome plant foods are also good sources of prebiotics, which act as food for the trillions of bacteria residing in your gut. An imbalance of friendly and unfriendly bacteria in the gut, known as *dysbiosis*, is thought to influence CKD progression by increasing inflammation. In addition to improving gut health, wholesome plant foods also help mitigate the acidosis that occurs as CKD progresses. By incorporating more wholesome plant foods in your diet, you neutralize the acid buildup and enhance the health of your gut, which, in turn, will improve the health of your kidneys.

WHY FIVE-INGREDIENT RECIPES?

Dealing with a chronic illness is burdensome enough without also feeling burdened by complicated, time-consuming recipes! Five-ingredient recipes make cooking for the renal diet a simple and enjoyable experience. When you only have to work with five ingredients, you spend less time shopping, prepping, and cleaning up. You may also enjoy savings on your grocery bill. My goal is that these recipes not only improve your condition, but also take the stress out of preparing meals for you and your family.

RENAL DIET GUIDELINES

An individualized renal diet works in various ways to support your remaining kidney function. This section reviews the renal diet guidelines, focusing on the nutrients that you may need to limit, as well as pointers to help you make smart choices for managing your CKD. The stage of your CKD, your individual lab values, and your other coexisting conditions are all important factors to consider. Before making dietary changes, always consult with your healthcare provider (HCP), who may provide you with more specific recommendations based on your unique health situation.

Potassium

Managing potassium can sometimes be confusing because intake recommendations change as CKD progresses. When we eat potassium, an electrolyte essential for many bodily functions, our body uses what is needed and excretes what is not. When kidney function declines as CKD progresses, the kidneys become less efficient at removing potassium through the urine. Potassium can build up in the blood when it isn't excreted properly, leading to a potentially dangerous condition called hyperkalemia. This is more likely to occur in the later stages of CKD.

In CKD stages 1 to 3, most people retain the ability to excrete excess potassium, which makes a potassium restriction unnecessary. Many plant foods are rich in potassium. According to the *British Journal of Medicine*, high dietary potassium intake is linked with a lowered risk of stroke and hypertension.

Since eating potassium-rich foods has been shown to be beneficial and since many people with CKD can still excrete potassium effectively, the most recent renal nutritional guidelines recommend that dietary potassium be adjusted to maintain a potassium blood level within the normal range. You should only restrict potassium if your HCP determines it necessary to maintain a potassium level within the normal range. See the Food Lists for the Renal Diet (page 153) for various foods' potassium content.

Protein

According to a thorough systematic review published in 2018 by the *Journal of the Academy of Nutrition and Dietetics*, current evidence suggests that people with CKD who lower their protein consumption may be able to slow CKD progression and improve their overall longevity and quality of life.

I tell my patients to think of lowering their dietary protein intake as a way of giving their kidneys a rest. Since kidneys process protein, eating too much of it can overtax them. When you're dealing with sick kidneys, the last thing you want to do is give them more work! In CKD, decreasing dietary protein intake has been shown to improve certain physical measures of the condition, such as protein in the urine.

Like potassium, protein is a nutrient that requires a lot of individualization, so determining how much is too much will depend on your stage of CKD, your height, and your unique health situation. The Protein section in Food Lists for the Renal Diet (page 153) table will help you estimate your daily protein needs, and as always, you should consult with your HCP for additional guidance.

If you need to lower your protein consumption, a plant-based diet is one of the easiest ways to achieve this. Most plant-based foods contain less protein than animal-derived foods, so moving toward a plant-based diet is an easy way to reduce the amount of protein in your diet without feeling like you are missing out. A plant-based diet is not necessarily a vegetarian or vegan diet. While some people with CKD may choose to become vegetarians or vegans, this approach may not be desirable or achievable for everyone. This cookbook advocates a plant-based diet that still includes animal-derived foods, but in smaller portions and less frequently, such as at one meal per day.

If you are on dialysis and need to increase the amount of protein you eat, chances are you won't need to make significant changes to your current diet. The standard American diet already contains more protein than The Dietary

Reference Intake recommends. Getting enough protein may become tricky, however, if you are experiencing a decreased appetite or unpleasant symptoms, such as nausea or fatigue. These issues can crop up in CKD's later stages and can make eating and preparing meals more challenging. Malnutrition is a common concern for many dialysis patients, and this can negatively impact quality of life and prognosis. A renal dietitian can help you manage these issues and may help you address them by prescribing certain dietary changes or nutrition supplements.

Phosphorus

Phosphorus is a mineral found in many different foods. Our bodies need a certain amount of phosphorus every day, and anything extra is removed through the urine. As CKD progresses and kidney function declines, the kidneys become less efficient at excreting extra dietary phosphorus in the urine.

Managing phosphorus intake is essential during every CKD stage to prevent serious renal complications, such as renal bone disease (weak and brittle bones) and cardiovascular disease. When it comes to managing dietary phosphorus, the source matters. There are three different sources of phosphorus in the diet: (1) plant-protein foods, such as whole grains, legumes, and nuts; (2) animal-protein foods, such as meat, cheese, and fish; and (3) phosphorus additives, which is the phosphorus added to processed foods and beverages, such as canned and bottled drinks, frozen meals, and many other packaged foods. See the Phosphorus section in Food Lists for the Renal Diet (page 153) table for guidance on how to look for phosphorus additives and preservatives in foods and beverages.

The source of phosphorus is important because, depending on the source, your body's ability to absorb it can vary tremendously. This variability in nutrient absorption is called bioavailability. The more bioavailable the phosphorus is in a food, the more you absorb. When someone has CKD and consumes a lot of bioavailable phosphorus, they are at greater risk of experiencing the negative complications associated with phosphorus.

The simplest way to manage your intake of dietary phosphorus is to understand what food sources contain the most bioavailable form of phosphorus and what sources contain the least. Estimates suggest that our bodies absorb as little as 10 percent of plant-protein-based phosphorous and as much as 100 percent of phosphorus additives. The absorption of the natural phosphorus found in animal foods such as meat and dairy is estimated to be somewhere between 40 and 60 percent. When it comes to phosphorus bioavailability, phosphorus additives found in processed foods are clearly the worst offenders.

Eating an abundance of plant foods, a moderate amount of animal foods, and as little phosphorus additives as possible will help you keep your phosphorus level in check. Phosphorus control tends to be the most challenging for people on dialysis because, at this stage, the kidney's ability to excrete phosphorus is greatly impaired. Additionally, people on dialysis sometimes need to increase their intake of higher phosphorus animal foods, such as meat and dairy, to meet their daily protein requirements. Many people on dialysis benefit from a medication, called a phosphorus binder, to help keep their phosphorus level under control. See the Phosphorus section in Food Lists for the Renal Diet (page 153) for more information.

Sodium

Sodium, a mineral and electrolyte obtained through diet, can contribute to high blood pressure when consumed in excessive amounts. High blood pressure increases the risk of cardiovascular disease and stroke, which is a major concern for people living with CKD. Blood pressure tends to increase as CKD progresses, and as a result, people with more advanced CKD tend to be the most salt sensitive. Limiting your sodium intake may help delay CKD progression even if your blood pressure is under control. According to a 2018 review of randomized control trial studies published in the journal *Nutrients*, moderate salt restriction significantly reduces protein in the urine, a major marker of kidney damage.

The recommended sodium intake for people with any stage of CKD is 2,300 milligrams per day. This is equal to about 1 teaspoon of salt. While this may seem like a lot, most Americans take in twice this amount daily, mainly in the form of "hidden salt." Hidden salt refers to the salt that is added to processed food and many restaurant foods. It is the salt that people are less aware of, since they aren't adding it in consciously during cooking or at the table. Hidden salt accounts for the majority of dietary sodium. According to the American Heart Association, processed food and many restaurant foods make up 71 percent of Americans' sodium intake. Salt added while cooking accounts for 6 percent, and salt at the table a mere 5 percent. By being mindful about the high sodium content in processed foods and many restaurant foods, you can keep your sodium intake within the recommended levels.

How can you become more mindful about sodium? You can start by habitually checking the sodium on nutrition labels before purchasing. Look for low-sodium or no-salt-added canned, frozen, jarred, and packaged foods. When dining out, be vocal about your low-sodium dietary needs. Many meals can be prepared with no salt or minimal salt. Your server can guide you toward the choices that will best fit your needs. See the Sodium section in Food Lists for the Renal Diet (page 153) to see a list of the sodium content in common foods.

High-Fiber Carbohydrates

When thinking about carbohydrates, it's helpful to group them into two different types: refined carbohydrates and unrefined carbohydrates. Refined carbohydrates include food and beverages such as sugar-sweetened drinks, pastries, white bread, and candy. Unrefined carbohydrates include vegetables, fruit, legumes, and whole grains. When refined carbohydrates predominate your diet, the risk of inflammation is higher, and inflammation can aggravate your CKD while also triggering other chronic health conditions such as obesity, diabetes, and cardiovascular disease. Unlike refined carbohydrates, unrefined carbohydrates provide a source of fiber in the diet. Consuming a high-fiber diet can create a good balance of healthy bacteria in the gut, which is beneficial for people with CKD.

While whole grains were traditionally discouraged on a renal diet, due to their higher potassium and phosphorus content, modern renal recommendations recognize the benefits of including them. Whole grains contain the least bioavailable form of phosphorus and are higher in fiber than refined grains. While there are certain exceptions, most whole grains provide only a marginal amount of extra potassium compared to refined grains. See the High-Fiber Foods section in Food Lists for the Renal Diet (page 153) for examples of high-fiber carbohydrates.

Heart-Healthy Fats

Let's be clear about one thing: The renal diet is not a low-fat diet. Don't think of fat as the enemy; instead, think of heart-healthy fat as your friend! Healthy fat adds rich flavor to your cooking and is also beneficial to your health.

Olive oil is a type of monounsaturated fat. It is one of the healthiest fats you can eat. According to a study published in the journal *BMC Medicine*, olive oil consumption is associated with a lower risk of developing cardiovascular disease. Compared to the general population, people with CKD are at a much higher risk of developing cardiovascular disease. With this in mind, don't be afraid to use olive oil liberally in your cooking and meal preparation. Avocado oil is another example of a monounsaturated fat. It is a popular cooking choice due to its high smoke point and mild flavor. Other heart-healthy fats include the fats found in certain fish such as salmon and mackerel, along with the heart-healthy fats found in nut butters, such as almond or peanut butter.

The primary dietary fats you'll want to avoid are the trans fats. Trans fats are found in processed foods that contain partially hydrogenated oil. (Look for this in the ingredients section on the nutrition label.) The American Heart Association recommends avoiding trans fats, as research links their consumption to a higher risk of developing heart disease and stroke. When it comes to saturated fats, found in foods such as butter, coconut oil, and cheese, the research is not as clear. While eating saturated fat has been shown to increase LDL (bad cholesterol), the link between saturated fat and the risk of heart disease remains unproven and hotly debated. If you have CKD and your cholesterol is under control, there is no reason to strictly eliminate saturated fats from your diet. It is much more important to focus on the more relevant nutrients to your condition, as mentioned in the previous sections. However, if you do struggle with an elevated LDL, you may need to be more careful about your saturated fat consumption. As always, consult with your HCP for further guidance on this topic.

Fluid Intake

Fluid needs are highly individual. If you have CKD stage 1 to 3, you may need to consume extra fluids to ensure that your kidneys stay adequately hydrated. If you have CKD stage 4 or 5, you may need to limit your fluid intake to prevent fluid retention. Speak with your HCP about how much fluid you should consume daily. Measuring your fluid intake is the best way to ensure you are meeting your body's needs.

STAGE-BY-STAGE NUTRITIONAL NEEDS

In 2018, the Academy of Nutrition and Dietetics and the National Kidney Foundation collaborated to merge, expand, and update the Kidney Disease Outcomes Quality Initiative (KDOQI) Nutrition Guidelines and the

2010 Evidence Analysis Library CKD Guidelines. The new guidelines are based on the highest-quality renal nutrition research available. Included in the guidelines are recommendations for protein, potassium, phosphorus, and sodium intake for CKD stages 3 to 5 and dialysis. The table Stage-by-Stage Nutritional Needs (page 11) provides a breakdown of the nutrition recommendations for each stage of CKD. Since the guideline did not specify what the recommendations are for stage 1 and 2 CKD, the recommendations included in the table for protein and sodium are based on the dietary guidelines given to the general population.

The Ideal Body Weight table provides an estimation of a person's ideal body weight based on height. This weight can be used to calculate your daily estimated protein needs. Please note that while the weights listed in this table can help provide a quick estimate of your lean body mass, they should be used with caution because many factors, such as genetics or muscle mass, can affect what a person's ideal body weight actually is. Your ideal body weight may be higher or lower than the weight listed in this table. As always, you should consult your HCP for more specific guidance.

Stage-by-Stage Nutritional Needs

CKD STAGE	PROTEIN	SODIUM	POTASSIUM	PHOSPHORUS
1–2	0.8 grams protein per kilogram of ideal body weight	2,300 milligrams per day for all stages	Adjust intake to maintain a blood potassium level within the normal range.	Adjust intake to maintain a blood phosphorus level within the normal range.
3–5 (non-dialysis)	0.55–0.6 grams protein per kilogram of ideal body weight			
Stage 5 Dialysis (all modalities)	1–1.2 grams protein per kilogram of ideal body weight			

FOR DIABETES

If you have diabetes and you have CKD stage 1–5 (not on dialysis), your protein needs are 0.8–0.9 grams per kilogram of ideal body weight.

If you are on dialysis and have diabetes, your protein needs are the same as non-diabetics (1–1.2 grams protein per kilogram of ideal body weight).

ADDITIONAL NOTES

Protein: To calculate your estimated protein needs, find your ideal body weight in the following table and multiply it by the grams of protein prescribed for your stage.

Example: If you are a male and 5 ft 8 with CKD stage 2, your ideal body weight is 70 kilograms. You would calculate your estimated daily protein needs by multiplying 0.8 grams protein by 70 kilograms.

$$0.8g \text{ protein x } 70 \text{ kilograms} = 56 \text{ grams protein per day.}$$

Sodium: Consuming less than 1,500 milligrams is not recommended as it may increase the risk of complications.

Ideal Body Weight

MALES		FEMALES	
HEIGHT	IBW (KG)	HEIGHT	IBW (KG)
5 ft	48	4 ft 10	41
5 ft 1	51	4 ft 11	43
5 ft 2	54	5 ft 0	45
5 ft 3	56	5 ft 1	48
5 ft 4	59	5 ft 2	50
5 ft 5	62	5 ft 3	52
5 ft 6	64	5 ft 4	54
5 ft 7	67	5 ft 5	57
5 ft 8	70	5 ft 6	59
5 ft 9	73	5 ft 7	61
5 ft 10	75	5 ft 8	64
5 ft 11	78	5 ft 9	66
6 ft	81	5 ft 10	68
6 ft 1	83	5 ft 11	70
6 ft 2	86	6 ft 0	73
6 ft 3	89		
6 ft 4	92		

IBW Table Disclaimer

Protein needs are calculated by multiplying your estimated weight on the chart in kilograms by a set amount of grams of protein. The renal nutrition guidelines recommend using ideal body weight instead of actual body weight when doing this calculation. Since being overweight or underweight is common among people with CKD, using actual weight to calculate protein needs could lead to overestimation or underestimation of a person's protein needs. The IBW chart provides a rough approximation of your lean body mass, which can be used in the protein calculation. For a more accurate estimation, consult with your HCP.

HOW TO READ NUTRITIONAL LABELS

Nutrition labels are a useful tool for choosing foods suitable for your health and personal needs. Below is a guide to help you read them.

Ingredients: Scan the list of ingredients before looking at the nutritional facts panel. Is there anything unexpected that catches your eye? For example, in a can of lentil soup, are there ingredients beyond just lentils, vegetables, and seasonings? Look for strange sounding additives, as this can be a red flag. Some additives, such as citric acid, are fine because they are used to help keep foods shelf-stable. Foods with a long list of additives, however, suggest that the food is highly processed. People with CKD need to be extra cautious of phosphorus additives, which are added to many processed foods to increase palatability and shelf life. Phosphorus additives are commonly added to baked goods, soda, enhanced meat products, and many other canned, bottled, and packaged foods. Phosphorus additives are the most bioavailable form of phosphorus in the diet. Below are examples of the most commonly used phosphorus additives by the food industry:

- Phosphoric acid
- Polyphosphate
- Sodium tripolyphosphate
- Tricalcium phosphate
- Trisodium phosphate

Serving Size: The nutrition information on the label reflects the serving size. If you eat more or less than the serving size, the nutrients will need to be adjusted accordingly. For example, if the serving size is 10 crackers and you eat 20 crackers, you will need to double all the nutrients to get the accurate nutrition information.

Nutrition Facts Panel: There is a lot of information on the nutrition facts panel, and some of the information will be more important to you based on your personal needs. People with CKD should check out the following nutrients:

- **Sodium:** The daily recommended amount of sodium for people with CKD is 2,300 milligrams. Think of this amount as your daily sodium budget. Every time you eat something containing sodium, you are spending some of your budget. It is important to be vigilant about checking the sodium content of processed and packaged foods.

- **Protein:** Daily protein needs are estimated based on weight. Being informed of your individual needs (see page 156) will allow you to quickly glance at a nutrition label and determine how the food fits into your daily protein allowance.

- **Fiber:** Fiber is the indigestible portion of plant foods found in vegetables, fruits, legumes, and whole grains. There are multiple benefits to consuming fiber, and many people do not consume enough. Men should aim to consume 38 grams of fiber daily, and women should aim to consume 25 grams of fiber daily.

- **Carbohydrates:** The Total Carbohydrate section of the label is helpful if you have diabetes and are counting carbs. Fiber, listed below it, is an indigestible carbohydrate that does not affect blood sugar levels, so it can be subtracted from the total carbs, providing you with the net carbohydrates of a given food.

- **Sugar:** Many patients I work with find it helpful to know that 4 grams of sugar equals 1 teaspoon of sugar. Using this number, if a product has 16 grams of sugar, you can easily calculate that it has 4 teaspoons of sugar. The American Heart Association recommends that men consume no more than 9 teaspoons of added sugar daily and that women consume no more than 6 teaspoons daily.

- **Potassium:** Potassium content will be listed on all nutrition labels by 2021, but until then, the easiest way to determine if a food contains high levels of potassium is to look at the ingredients. Look for high-potassium ingredients (see the Potassium section in Food Lists for the Renal Diet on page 153) and remember that ingredients on food labels are listed by quantity used, from greatest to least.

YOUR FIRST SHOPPING TRIP: MAKE SIX EASY MEALS

Planning your meals ahead of time creates structure and makes it more likely that you will stick to the renal diet. When thinking about what you want to prepare and eat in the days ahead, it's helpful to choose meals with similar ingredients, as this will allow you to cut down on food waste and cost. The recipes in this book contain several ingredients that are used in multiple recipes. With just 27 ingredients, you can make the following six recipes from the book:

1. Overnight Cranberry Almond Oats (Breakfast)
2. Red Beans and Rice (Entrée)
3. Fish Taco Filling (Entrée)
4. Hearty Veggie Stew (Entrée)
5. Italian-Inspired Rice and Peas (Side)
6. **Almond-Cranberry Cookies (Dessert)**

Shopping List

PRODUCE

Baby carrots (1 [16-ounce] bag)

Cabbage coleslaw mix with carrots (1 [16-ounce] bag)

Celery (1 bunch)

Lime (1)

Onions, yellow (2)

Shallots (2)

Sweet potato, large (1)

CANNED GOODS

Kidney beans, no salt added (1 [15-ounce] can)

Vegetable broth, low-sodium (3 cups)

PANTRY

Almond butter

Black pepper, freshly ground

Brown rice (1 cup)

Brown sugar

Chili powder

Corn tortillas (4)

Cranberries, dried,
unsweetened (if available)
(1 ½ cups)

Mint leaves, dried

Oats, old-fashioned,
rolled (4 cups)

Olive oil, extra-virgin

Salt

Vanilla extract

Baby peas (2 [12-ounce] bags)

Bell pepper and onion blend
(1 [12-ounce] bag)

Almond milk, unsweetened
(16 ounces)

Parmesan cheese, grated (½ ounce)

Egg (1)

Sole (3 [6-ounce] fillets)

BASIC KITCHEN EQUIPMENT

In addition to a cutting board, these are the basic equipment pieces that you'll need to make this book's recipes. The recipes try to account for various cooking methods if you don't have one of these items, such as how to cook a recipe in the oven if you don't have a slow cooker.

Cast-iron skillet   A cast-iron skillet is naturally nonstick without relying on the use of Teflon. It's best to avoid Teflon because it contains a chemical that is considered to be "likely carcinogenic." A cast-iron skillet can be used on the stove as well as in the oven. Because a cast iron skillet is made of iron, some of the iron from the skillet is released into your food during the cooking process. Many people with CKD stand to benefit from an iron boost, as iron deficiency anemia is a common problem, especially for people on dialysis.

Food processor   A food processor has the ability to mix, shred, blend, grind, slice, and chop a wide variety of foods. Due to its wide range of functions, a food processor would be an excellent addition to any kitchen.

Food storage containers   Equipping your kitchen with several food storage containers will allow you to store leftovers for later use or to cook in bulk. Ideally, look for non-plastic containers, as plastic can leach harmful chemicals into your food, especially when heated. Glass, stainless steel, or silicone-based containers are all good alternatives.

Knives   When it comes to food preparation, every cook will tell you how essential it is to have a decent set of knives. The quality matters with knives, so if you can afford to splurge a little, know that the investment will serve you for years to come. If you can't afford a whole set, purchase a good chef's knife, as this can be used to slice and dice pretty much any kind of food.

Meat thermometer   A meat thermometer helps ensure that meat, poultry, and fish are cooked to a safe temperature every time. Look for an instant-read thermometer so that you can obtain a reading in seconds.

Slow cooker A slow cooker cooks food slowly without slowing you down! When you are busy, it can be hard to allocate the time to cook a meal. A slow cooker is a great solution to this problem. Most slow cooker recipes have you add all the ingredients needed at one time. After you've added the ingredients, you simply adjust the slow cooker to the appropriate setting and let it run for a number of hours (usually 4 to 8). Your meal will be waiting for you when you return!

5 TIPS AND TRICKS TO MAKE THINGS EVEN EASIER

These five tips and tricks will help your kitchen run even more smoothly:

Cook in bulk. Making enough food to have leftovers is something every cook should get into the habit of doing. In addition to reducing the amount of time you spend cooking each week, some people even notice that food tastes better when it's a couple of days old. This is probably because the flavors have had a chance to marinate. Store leftovers in the refrigerator for up to three to four days or freeze them and use within three to four months.

Get the right tools. The right tools help make cooking a safe and efficient process. Essential tools include a sharp knife, measuring cups, measuring spoons, and cutting boards.

Organize your work and storage spaces. Don't you hate it when you know you bought an ingredient, but you can't find it anywhere? Clutter and a lack of organization in the kitchen can detract from the enjoyment and convenience of cooking, so be sure to put some time into keeping your pantry, refrigerator, and freezer in order so that items are easy to find and accessible. A spice rack is great for organizing spices. Try mounting one on the wall; you can even put the spices in alphabetical order. There are many other ways to organize your kitchen better. Consider drawer dividers or cabinet standing dividers, so that cookware and other kitchen items are easy to access.

Prep your five ingredients. Before you start cooking, measure out and prepare all the ingredients you'll need for a recipe. Getting this step out of the way will allow you to focus solely on cooking.

Make use of convenient ingredients. Many ingredients can be purchased ready to go, reducing the amount of time needed to prepare them. For example, vegetables can be purchased precut (fresh or frozen), and beans can be purchased canned. Always make sure that the prepared foods you buy are minimally processed with no added salt.

ABOUT THE RECIPES

The book's recipes require 5 ingredients (excluding salt, pepper, oil, and water) and help make following the renal diet as simple as possible. As you cook your way through the book, you'll notice there are tips to vary the herbs and spices in these recipes. All the recipes contain a low to moderate amount of sodium, potassium, and phosphorus, making them suitable for all stages of CKD. In addition to containing nutritional information, each recipe contains at least one recipe label and one recipe tip. Recipe labels include:

Low Protein: Recipes with this label have less than 15 grams of protein per serving in larger dishes such as entrées, and less than 5 grams of protein per serving in smaller dishes such as snacks and desserts. If your estimated protein needs fall between 30 and 40 grams per day, you should choose mostly low-protein recipes.

Medium Protein: Recipes with this label have protein that ranges from 15 to 24 grams per serving in larger dishes such as entrées, and protein that ranges from 5 to 9 grams per serving in smaller dishes such as snacks and desserts. If your estimated protein needs fall between 40 and 60 grams per day, you should choose a combination of low- and medium-protein recipes.

High Protein: Recipes with this label have 25 or more grams of protein per serving in larger dishes such as entrées, and 10 or more grams of protein per serving in smaller dishes such as snacks and desserts. If your protein needs are 60 grams or more per day, choose a combination of medium- and high-protein recipes.

High Fiber: Recipes with this label have more than 5 grams of fiber per serving in larger dishes such as entrées, and more than 2 grams of fiber per serving in smaller dishes such as snacks and desserts.

Diabetes-Friendly: This label indicates that the recipe is good for people with diabetes or that it contains a tip on how to make it so.

Vegan/Vegetarian: Vegetarian recipes do not use any meat, poultry, or fish, but may use animal products like honey, milk, and butter. Recipes labeled as vegan contain no animal products.

Gluten-Free: These recipes contain no gluten using the ingredients listed. Always check ingredient packaging for gluten-free labeling.

Recipe tips include:

Make It Diabetes-Friendly Tip: Suggests a modification to make the recipe appropriate for people with diabetes.

Increase Protein Tip: Suggests a modification to increase the protein content of the recipe, which may make it more appropriate for people on dialysis or for someone who has higher protein needs due to their body size.

Reduce Protein Tip: Suggests a modification to reduce the protein content of the recipe, which may make it more appropriate for someone with CKD stages 3 to 5 (non-dialysis).

Make It Easier Tip: Suggests a modification to make the recipe more convenient to prepare.

Appliance Tip: Provides information on how to prepare a recipe if you don't have the appliance used in the recipe.

Ingredient Tip: Provides advice or guidance about the use of a specific ingredient in a recipe.

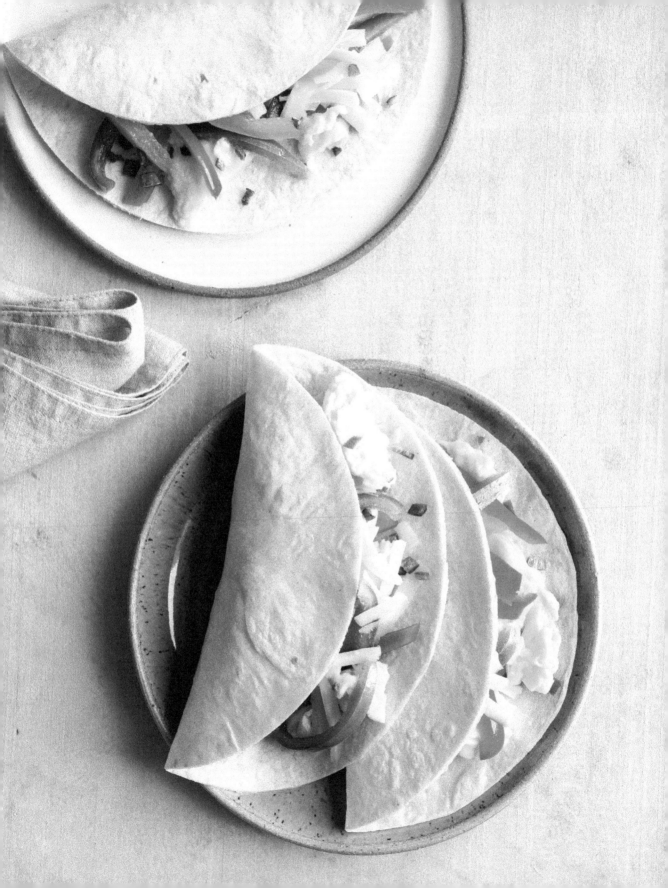

CHAPTER 2

Breakfast and Smoothies

⇐ *Breakfast Tacos, page 25*

Peanut Butter and Jelly Granola

LOW PROTEIN, VEGAN

Serves 6 / Prep Time: 15 minutes / Cook Time: 30 minutes

Granola is the perfect make-ahead breakfast recipe. This variation is full of fiber and tastes delicious. It combines peanut butter and jelly for a PB&J-like treat. Eat it plain or pair it with almond milk and some fruit for a nourishing breakfast bowl. It also makes a great yogurt parfait topping.

2 cups rolled oats

¼ cup peanut butter

3 tablespoons maple syrup

1 tablespoon water

½ teaspoon ground cinnamon

Pinch salt

¼ cup jelly, any flavor

1. Preheat the oven to 325°F. Line a rimmed baking sheet with parchment paper and set aside.

2. Pour the oats into a mixing bowl and set aside.

3. In a small saucepan, combine the peanut butter, maple syrup, water, cinnamon, and salt. Heat over low heat until the peanut butter is melted.

4. Pour the peanut butter mixture over the oats and toss to coat. Spread onto the baking sheet.

5. In a small bowl in the microwave or in a small pan on low heat, heat the jelly until it's thin, about 1 minute. Drizzle over the oat mixture on the baking sheet.

6. Bake for 20 to 30 minutes, stirring once during baking, until the granola is golden brown.

7. Cool completely and store in an airtight container at room temperature for up to a week.

Ingredient Tip: You can substitute sweetened dried cherries or cranberries for the jelly if you'd like. You can also use other nut or seed butters, such as almond butter or sunflower seed butter, in place of the peanut butter.

Per Serving (⅓ cup) Calories: 230; Total fat: 7g; Saturated fat: 1g; Sodium: 79mg; Phosphorus: 150mg; Potassium: 190mg; Carbohydrates: 37g; Fiber: 4g; Protein: 6g; Sugar: 14g

Breakfast Tacos

DIABETES-FRIENDLY, GLUTEN-FREE, LOW PROTEIN, VEGETARIAN

Serves 4 / Prep Time: 15 minutes / Cook Time: 15 minutes

Tacos are fun, easy, and versatile. They are perfect for any meal, and the possible filling combinations are endless—from just veggies to this egg version. These tacos have a bit of a kick thanks to jalapeño and pepper jack cheese. If spicy isn't your speed, you can omit the jalapeño pepper.

2 tablespoons extra-virgin olive oil

1½ cups frozen bell peppers

2 tablespoons water, divided

1 jalapeño pepper, minced

6 large eggs

⅛ teaspoon salt

⅛ teaspoon freshly ground
   black pepper

4 corn tortillas

½ cup shredded pepper jack cheese

1. In a medium skillet, heat the olive oil over medium heat.

2. Add the bell peppers and stir. Add 1 tablespoon of water and cover the pan. Cook for 3 to 4 minutes, or until the vegetables are thawed and hot. Add the jalapeño pepper and cook for about 1 minute.

3. While the vegetables are cooking, in a medium bowl, combine the eggs and the remaining 1 tablespoon of water and beat well.

4. Add the eggs to the skillet and cook for 4 to 6 minutes, stirring occasionally, until the eggs are set. Sprinkle with the salt and pepper.

5. Heat the tortillas as directed on the package. Make tacos with the tortillas, egg filling, and cheese and serve.

Ingredient Tip: To make this recipe vegan, replace the eggs with 2 cups of canned, low-sodium black beans and the pepper jack cheese with shredded vegan cheese. This substitution will increase the potassium to 510mg per serving.

Per Serving (1 taco) Calories: 283; Total fat: 19g; Saturated fat: 6g; Sodium: 252mg; Phosphorus: 259mg; Potassium: 262mg; Carbohydrates: 15g; Fiber: 2g; Protein: 13g; Sugar: 4g

Rice and Almond Hot Cereal

GLUTEN-FREE, HIGH FIBER, LOW PROTEIN, VEGAN

Serves 6 / Prep Time: 5 minutes / Cook Time: 7 hours

Want to wake up to a breakfast that's ready to go? This recipe is perfect for that. It's cooked overnight in a slow cooker, so you'll have a delicious and warm breakfast waiting for you in the morning. Top your bowl with some slivered almonds and enjoy your warm and hearty breakfast.

3 cups unsweetened almond milk

2 cups water

1½ cups wild rice, rinsed

1 cup brown rice

¼ cup maple syrup

⅛ teaspoon salt

⅔ cup slivered almonds, toasted

1. In a 3-quart slow cooker, combine the almond milk, water, wild rice, brown rice, maple syrup, and salt. Stir.

2. Cover and cook on low for 7 to 8 hours.

3. Top with the almonds and serve.

Appliance Tip: If you don't have a slow cooker, you can make this recipe on the stovetop. Combine the wild rice and brown rice with the almond milk, water, maple syrup, and salt in a heavy saucepan over medium-high heat and bring to a simmer. Reduce the heat to low and simmer for 30 to 35 minutes, stirring occasionally, until both types of rice are tender. Sprinkle with the almonds and serve.

Per Serving Calories: 377; Total fat: 9g; Saturated fat: 1g; Sodium: 140mg; Phosphorus: 339mg; Potassium: 443mg; Carbohydrates: 66g; Fiber: 5g; Protein: 11g; Sugar: 10g

Overnight Cranberry Almond Oats

HIGH FIBER, LOW PROTEIN, VEGAN

Serves 6 / Prep Time: 5 minutes

Cranberries are rich in phytonutrients, which are plant compounds with anti-inflammatory and antioxidant properties. Make sure to look for unsweetened cranberries because many sweetened varieties have up to 4 teaspoons of sugar per serving. The vanilla and almond butter will offset the cranberries' tartness, but feel free to sweeten the oats with a little honey or maple syrup. Overnight soaking will make the quick-cooking oats too soft, so be sure to use old-fashioned oats.

4 cups old-fashioned rolled oats

2 cups unsweetened almond milk

2 cups water

1 cup dried
   unsweetened cranberries

¼ cup almond butter

2 teaspoons vanilla extract

1. In a medium bowl, combine the oats, almond milk, water, cranberries, almond butter, and vanilla and mix well. It's okay if the almond butter doesn't mix completely with the other ingredients. Cover tightly with plastic wrap. Refrigerate overnight, or at least 6 hours.

2. When you're ready to eat, stir the mixture and serve. You can heat it if you'd like; just put it into a saucepan and heat over low heat until the cereal is steaming.

Ingredient Tip: This recipe can easily be made gluten-free. Just look for gluten-free rolled oats. Oats are naturally gluten-free but most commercial brands are contaminated with gluten during manufacturing. Gluten-free oats are produced in facilities that take care to avoid cross contamination.

Per Serving (¾ cup) Calories: 367; Total fat: 10g; Saturated fat: 1g; Sodium: 62mg; Phosphorus: 285mg; Potassium: 342mg; Carbohydrates: 61g; Fiber: 8g; Protein: 10g; Sugar: 3g

Turmeric, Bell Pepper, and Squash Omelet

DIABETES-FRIENDLY, GLUTEN-FREE, MEDIUM PROTEIN, VEGETARIAN

Serves 4 / Prep Time: 10 minutes / Cook Time: 10 minutes

This omelet's vibrant color is the first thing you'll notice. Turmeric provides the yellow color, a pleasant spiciness, and a multitude of health benefits. Research conducted on turmeric's potent anti-inflammatory powers shows its potential for improving cardiovascular, kidney, and gastrointestinal health. The bell pepper and yellow squash add fiber, texture, and flavor to the omelet.

---

2 tablespoons extra-virgin olive oil

½ teaspoon ground turmeric

1 yellow bell pepper, chopped

1 small yellow summer
  squash, chopped

8 large eggs

1 tablespoon water

Salt

Freshly ground black pepper

½ cup shredded Colby cheese

---

1. In a medium nonstick skillet, heat the olive oil over medium heat. Add the turmeric and stir for 30 seconds, until fragrant.

2. Add the bell pepper and squash and cook for 3 to 5 minutes, or until tender, stirring occasionally. Transfer the vegetables to a plate and set aside; do not drain or wipe out the skillet.

3. Meanwhile, in a small bowl, beat the eggs with the water, salt, and pepper until frothy and combined. Add the egg mixture to the skillet.

4. Cook for 5 to 7 minutes, running a spatula around the edges of the omelet to let the uncooked portion flow under the cooked eggs, and shaking the pan occasionally, until the eggs are just set.

5. Top half of the omelet with the vegetable mixture and sprinkle with the cheese. With a spatula, fold the omelet in half and serve.

Reduce Protein Tip: To make this a low-protein recipe, reduce the number of eggs to 6. The protein content will decrease to 14g per serving.

Per Serving Calories: 286; Total fat: 22g; Saturated fat: 7g; Sodium: 211mg; Phosphorus: 263mg; Potassium: 340mg; Carbohydrates: 5g; Fiber: 1g; Protein: 17g; Sugar: 4g

Baked Egg Omelet

DIABETES-FRIENDLY, GLUTEN-FREE, MEDIUM PROTEIN, VEGETARIAN

Serves 4 / Prep Time: 10 minutes / Cook Time: 35 minutes

A baked omelet may take more time, but it can be more convenient than standing at the stove waiting for your eggs to cook. The suggested vegetables in this recipe add fiber, color, and many vitamins and minerals. Feel free to swap out the vegetables in this dish for other types that you like. This omelet is also a good opportunity to use up any leftover cooked vegetables you have in your fridge.

Olive oil cooking spray

1½ cups frozen chopped broccoli, thawed and drained

1 cup frozen peas, thawed and drained

9 large eggs

2 tablespoons unsweetened almond milk

Salt

Freshly ground black pepper

½ cup shredded Monterey Jack cheese

1. Preheat the oven to 350°F. Spray a 9-inch square pan with cooking spray and set aside.

2. Place the broccoli and peas in the pan and distribute evenly.

3. In a medium bowl, beat the eggs with the almond milk, salt, and pepper. Pour over the vegetables in the pan.

4. Bake the omelet for 30 to 35 minutes or until it is puffed, light golden brown, and firm to the touch.

5. Remove the omelet from the oven and sprinkle with the cheese. Cover the pan with a plate and let stand for 2 minutes to melt the cheese, then serve.

Reduce Protein Tip: To make this a low-protein recipe, use 6 egg whites and 1 whole egg (instead of 9 whole eggs). The protein content will decrease to 14g per serving.

Per Serving Calories: 252; Total fat: 15g; Saturated fat: 6g; Sodium: 257mg; Phosphorus: 295mg; Potassium: 290mg; Carbohydrates: 10g; Fiber: 4g; Protein: 20g; Sugar: 4g

Banana Oat Pancakes

DIABETES-FRIENDLY, HIGH FIBER, LOW PROTEIN, VEGETARIAN

Serves 4 / Prep Time: 15 minutes / Cook Time: 25 minutes

Typical pancake ingredients include white flour, sugar, and maple syrup, making them more of a dessert than a breakfast. Instead of white flour, this recipe uses oats that are higher in fiber and other nutrients, and uses banana as a sweetener. Don't worry, despite including bananas, this recipe remains low in potassium. Only two bananas are used to make four servings.

⅓ cup rolled oats

4 large eggs

2 large ripe bananas

1 teaspoon vanilla extract

Pinch salt

2 tablespoons butter

1. In a food processor, place the oats and process until finely ground; set aside.

2. In a medium bowl, beat the eggs until light and lemon colored.

3. In another bowl, combine the ground oatmeal, bananas, vanilla, and salt and mix well.

4. Fold the eggs into the banana mixture until combined.

5. In a large nonstick skillet, melt the butter over medium heat.

6. Drop the batter onto the skillet in scant ¼-cup portions. Cook for 2 to 3 minutes or until the pancakes have small bubbles on the top and the edges look cooked. Flip the pancakes and cook for another 2 to 3 minutes on the second side. Serve.

Increase Protein Tip: To make this a medium-protein recipe, add 1 scoop (2 tablespoons) of unflavored or vanilla protein powder. Adding a protein powder with 30 grams of protein per scoop will increase the protein to 16g per serving.

Per Serving (2 pancakes) Calories: 217; Total fat: 12g; Saturated fat: 5g; Sodium: 148mg; Phosphorus: 130mg; Potassium: 334mg; Carbohydrates: 21g; Fiber: 8g; Protein: 8g; Sugar: 9g

Blueberry Scones

GLUTEN-FREE, LOW PROTEIN, VEGETARIAN

Serves 8 / Prep Time: 20 minutes / Cook Time: 25 minutes

Looking for a delicious breakfast treat to serve for brunch? This recipe calls for a gluten-free flour blend. Look for a flour blend that contains nutrient-dense ingredients. Many are made with white rice flour, making them no better a choice than regular white flour. Bob's Red Mill makes a gluten-free all-purpose baking flour that contains fava bean, sorghum, and chickpea flour. Using this flour makes for a higher-fiber, more nutritious scone.

2 cups gluten-free flour mix
or blend
¼ cup brown sugar
2 teaspoons baking powder
¼ teaspoon salt

½ cup water
5 tablespoons extra-virgin olive oil
1 large egg
⅔ cup fresh blueberries

1. Preheat the oven to 375°F. Line a baking sheet with parchment paper and set aside.
2. In a large bowl, combine the flour mix, brown sugar, baking powder, and salt and mix well.
3. In a small bowl, beat the water, olive oil, and egg until combined.
4. Add the egg mixture to the flour mixture all at once and stir, just until a dough forms. Gently work in the blueberries with your hands.
5. On the prepared baking sheet, form the mixture into an 8-inch circle. Cut into 8 wedges and separate the wedges slightly.
6. Bake the scones for 20 to 25 minutes or until light golden brown. Remove from the baking sheet and cool on a wire rack before serving.

Ingredient Tip: You can make this recipe with any fruit. Try using fresh raspberries or chopped strawberries. Other good choices include dried fruits such as dried cranberries or raisins.

Per Serving (1 scone) Calories: 218; Total fat: 10g; Saturated fat: 1g; Sodium: 206mg; Phosphorus: 108mg; Potassium: 167mg; Carbohydrates: 31g; Fiber: 3g; Protein: 4g; Sugar: 9g

Crunchy Granola Yogurt Bowl

HIGH FIBER, LOW PROTEIN, VEGETARIAN

Serves 4 / Prep Time: 10 minutes

A thick and creamy yogurt pairs perfectly with granola's satisfying crunch. Look for plain whole-milk yogurt because flavored selections tend to contain a lot of sugar. If purchasing a granola, look for a brand that has less than 5 grams of sugar per serving, such as some varieties of the KIND brand. Alternatively, you can make your own Peanut Butter and Jelly Granola (page 24).

3 cups plain whole-milk yogurt
1½ teaspoons vanilla extract
1 cup granola

½ cup dried raisins
½ cup chopped pecans

1. In a medium bowl, combine the yogurt and vanilla.
2. Into glasses or small bowls, layer the yogurt with the granola, raisins, and pecans. Serve.

Ingredient Tip: You can use any type of dried fruit or nuts in this recipe. Try unsweetened dried cherries, blueberries, or goji berries, or substitute walnuts or macadamia nuts for the sliced pecans.

Per Serving (¾ cup) Calories: 360; Total fat: 17g; Saturated fat: 5g; Sodium: 119mg; Phosphorus: 230mg; Potassium: 478mg; Carbohydrates: 44g; Fiber: 4g; Protein: 10g; Sugar: 24g

Slow Cooker Steel-Cut Oats

HIGH FIBER, LOW PROTEIN, VEGAN

Serves 4 / Prep Time: 10 minutes / Cook Time: 7 hours

Steel-cut oats are oats that are cut into pieces, instead of being steamed and rolled through mills like rolled oats. When cooked, they have a firmer and chewier texture—even when prepared in a slow cooker. They also have a lower glycemic index compared to regular oats. You can serve these with maple syrup, fresh fruit, chopped nuts, or chia seeds.

3½ cups water

3 cups unsweetened almond milk

1½ cups steel-cut oats

2 tablespoons honey

1 tablespoon vanilla extract

1 teaspoon ground cinnamon

1. In a 3-quart slow cooker, combine the water, almond milk, oats, honey, vanilla, and cinnamon and stir.

2. Cover and cook on low for 7 to 8 hours. Serve.

Appliance Tip: If you don't have a 3-quart slow cooker, you can simmer all the ingredients in a pan on the stovetop, set on medium-low, for about 20 minutes or until the oats are tender but still slightly firm.

Per Serving (¾ cup) Calories: 298; Total fat: 6g; Saturated fat: 1g; Sodium: 132mg; Phosphorus: 265mg; Potassium: 351mg; Carbohydrates: 51g; Fiber: 6g; Protein: 9g; Sugar: 10g

Peach Melba Smoothie

GLUTEN-FREE, LOW PROTEIN, VEGETARIAN

Serves 4 / Prep Time: 10 minutes

Smoothies are a great way to make breakfast in a hurry, but with many recipes calling for sweeteners and fruit juice, smoothies often end up being more like a dessert. This recipe uses whole fruit without any fruit juice or sweetener. The raspberries and peaches provide fiber and flavor.

2 cups frozen peach slices

1½ cups plain whole-milk yogurt

1 cup frozen raspberries

1 cup ice cubes

1 tablespoon freshly squeezed lemon juice

1 teaspoon vanilla extract

1. In a food processor or heavy-duty blender, combine the peaches, yogurt, raspberries, ice, lemon juice, and vanilla and blend until smooth.

2. Pour into glasses and serve.

Ingredient Tip: To make this recipe vegan, you can use plain coconut yogurt. It adds a nice creaminess and coconut flavor along with blood-sugar-balancing fat. Adding a tablespoon of chia seeds to your smoothie will make it high in fiber and extra filling.

Per Serving Calories: 126; Total fat: 4g; Saturated fat: 2g; Sodium: 49mg; Phosphorus: 119mg; Potassium: 389mg; Carbohydrates: 20g; Fiber: 4g; Protein: 2g; Sugar: 11g

Strawberry Spice Smoothie

GLUTEN-FREE, LOW PROTEIN, VEGETARIAN

Serves 4 / Prep Time: 10 minutes

Strawberries provide a blast of vitamin C in this easy smoothie recipe. The nutmeg and ginger add a hint of spice and the Greek yogurt base makes this smoothie creamy and full of protein. Using a plant-based yogurt such as coconut or almond milk–based yogurt would lower the protein without sacrificing the creamy consistency.

2 cups frozen strawberries

1½ cups plain whole-milk
  Greek yogurt

1 cup ice

2 tablespoons chia seeds

⅛ teaspoon ground nutmeg

¼ teaspoon ground ginger

1. In a food processor or blender, combine the strawberries, yogurt, ice, chia seeds, nutmeg, and ginger and process until smooth.

2. Pour into glasses and serve.

Increase Protein Tip: To make this a medium-protein recipe, add 2 scoops of unflavored or vanilla protein powder. The protein content will increase to 20g per serving.

Per Serving Calories: 153; Total fat: 7g; Saturated fat: 4g; Sodium: 64mg; Phosphorus: 158mg; Potassium: 372mg; Carbohydrates: 18g; Fiber: 4g; Protein: 5g; Sugar: 11g

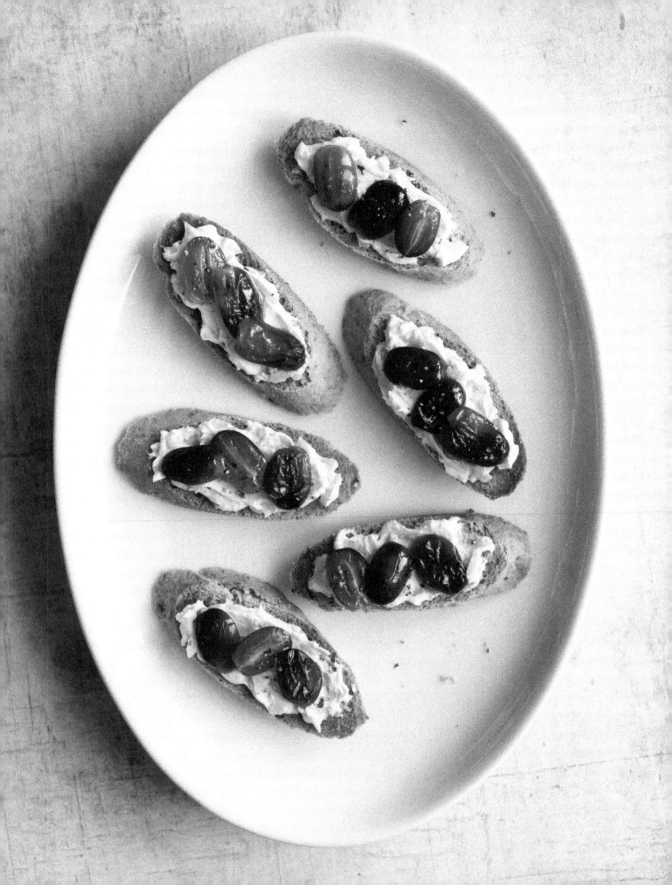

CHAPTER 3

Sides and Snacks

Cabbage Apple Stir-Fry   38

Parmesan Roasted Cauliflower   39

Celery and Fennel Salad with Cranberries   40

Kale with Caramelized Onions   41

Italian-Inspired Rice and Peas   42

Baked Jicama Fries   43

Double-Boiled Sweet Potatoes   44

Roasted Onion Dip   45

Roasted Garlic White Bean Dip   46

Green Goddess Dip   48

Crab and Carrot Dip   49

Roasted Grape Crostini   50

⇦Roasted Grape Crostini, page 50

37

Cabbage Apple Stir-Fry

DIABETES-FRIENDLY, GLUTEN-FREE, HIGH FIBER, LOW PROTEIN, VEGAN

Serves 4 / Prep Time: 15 minutes / Cook Time: 10 minutes

Fruit and vegetables are delicious when paired together, but an unexpected example might be the tasty combination of cabbage and apples. Red cabbage's nutty, slightly sweet flavor is enhanced by the addition of tart Granny Smith apples. Caraway seeds add a hint of spice to the recipe. If you don't have caraway seeds, you can substitute dill seeds or fennel seeds. This recipe is as vibrant in color as it is delicious.

2 tablespoons extra-virgin olive oil

3 cups chopped red cabbage

2 tablespoons water

1 Granny Smith apple, chopped

3 scallions, both white and green parts, chopped

1 tablespoon freshly squeezed lemon juice

1 teaspoon caraway seeds

Pinch salt

1. In a large skillet or wok, heat the olive oil over medium-high heat.

2. Add the cabbage and stir-fry for 2 minutes. Add the water, cover, and cook for 2 minutes.

3. Uncover and stir in the apple and scallions and sprinkle with the lemon juice, caraway seeds, and salt. Stir-fry for 4 to 6 minutes longer, or until the cabbage is crisp-tender. Serve.

Make It Easier: You can use pre-shredded cabbage in this recipe; just omit the water and add the apples and scallions to the skillet at the same time.

Per Serving Calories: 106; Total fat: 7g; Saturated fat: 1g; Sodium: 55mg; Phosphorus: 27mg; Potassium: 206mg; Carbohydrates: 11g; Fiber: 3g; Protein: 1g; Sugar: 7g

Parmesan Roasted Cauliflower

DIABETES-FRIENDLY, GLUTEN-FREE, MEDIUM PROTEIN, VEGETARIAN

Serves 4 / Prep Time: 15 minutes / Cook Time: 25 minutes

Cauliflower is one of the healthiest foods you can eat. A member of the cruciferous vegetable family, cauliflower is high in fiber as well as anti-inflammatory antioxidants and phytonutrients. If you've only ever tasted cauliflower boiled, you'll love the delicious texture of cauliflower when it is roasted. The Parmesan cheese and garlic contribute excellent flavor. To make this recipe vegan, omit the Parmesan and replace with ½ cup of nutritional yeast.

4 cups cauliflower florets

½ cup grated Parmesan cheese

2 tablespoons extra-virgin olive oil

4 garlic cloves, minced

½ teaspoon dried thyme leaves

¼ teaspoon freshly ground
  black pepper

⅛ teaspoon salt

1. Preheat the oven to 400°F.

2. On a baking sheet, combine the cauliflower, Parmesan cheese, olive oil, garlic, thyme, pepper, and salt and toss to coat.

3. Roast for 25 to 30 minutes, stirring once during cooking time, until the cauliflower has light golden brown edges and is tender. Serve.

Make It Easier Tip: You can often buy cauliflower that is already cut into florets in the grocery store. Look for florets that are pure white with no dark spots or areas, as those indicate a less fresh vegetable.

Per Serving Calories: 144; Total fat: 11g; Saturated fat: 3g; Sodium: 332mg; Phosphorus: 130mg; Potassium: 359mg; Carbohydrates: 4g; Fiber: 1g; Protein: 6g; Sugar: 2g

Celery and Fennel Salad with Cranberries

GLUTEN-FREE, LOW PROTEIN, VEGAN

Serves 6 / Prep Time: 15 minutes

While celery is a common salad ingredient, it's rarely the star. As the main ingredient in this recipe, celery contributes excellent crunch and a mild, earthy flavor. Fresh fennel provides additional texture along with a slight hint of licorice. Dried cranberries add a touch of sweetness and elegant color to this tasty, yet nutrient-dense recipe. Don't buy pretrimmed celery sticks; you need the whole head because this recipe uses the leaves too.

¼ cup extra-virgin olive oil

2 tablespoons freshly squeezed lemon juice

1 tablespoon Dijon mustard

2 cups sliced celery

½ cup chopped fennel

½ cup dried cranberries

2 tablespoons minced celery leaves

1. In a serving bowl, whisk the olive oil, lemon juice, and mustard.
2. Add the celery, fennel, and cranberries to the dressing and toss to coat. Sprinkle with the celery leaves and serve.

Diabetes-Friendly Tip: To make this recipe diabetes-friendly omit the dried cranberries from this salad as most varieties contain added sugar. You could substitute a few fresh, sliced strawberries instead.

Per Serving Calories: 130; Total fat: 9g; Saturated fat: 1g; Sodium: 88mg; Phosphorus: 13mg; Potassium: 107mg; Carbohydrates: 13g; Fiber: 1g; Protein: <1g; Sugar: 10g

Kale with Caramelized Onions

DIABETES-FRIENDLY, GLUTEN-FREE, HIGH FIBER, LOW PROTEIN, VEGETARIAN

Serves 4 / Prep Time: 15 minutes / Cook Time: 20 minutes

There are several kinds of kale on the market, and any variety will work for this recipe. Curly kale has very crinkled leaves, lacinato kale (aka dinosaur kale) has blue-green leaves, and baby kale has flat, green leaves. Kale is high in goitrogens, a plant compound that can disrupt the thyroid hormone. Cooking kale decreases these compounds, tenderizes the stiff leaves, and reduces the bitter flavor. Pairing it with caramelized onions creates a wonderful side dish.

1 yellow onion, chopped

2 tablespoons butter

1 tablespoon extra-virgin olive oil

1 bunch kale, rinsed and torn
    into pieces

2 tablespoons water

1 tablespoon freshly squeezed
    lemon juice

1 teaspoon maple syrup

Salt

Freshly ground black pepper

1. In a heavy saucepan, combine the onion, butter, and olive oil over medium heat. Cook for about 3 minutes, until the onion starts to become translucent, stirring frequently.

2. Reduce the heat to low and continue cooking for 10 to 15 minutes longer, stirring frequently, until the onion starts to brown.

3. Increase the heat to medium and add the kale and water. Cover the pan and cook for about 2 minutes, shaking the pan occasionally, until the kale starts to soften.

4. Add the lemon juice and maple syrup, and season with salt and pepper. Cook for 3 to 4 minutes longer, stirring frequently, until the kale is tender. Serve.

Appliance Tip: You can cook this recipe in a 4-quart slow cooker. Combine all the ingredients and stir. Cover the slow cooker and cook on low for 6 to 8 hours or until the onions and kale are tender. Stir and serve.

Per Serving Calories: 115; Total fat: 10g; Saturated fat: 4g; Sodium: 112mg; Phosphorus: 37mg; Potassium: 224mg; Carbohydrates: 6g; Fiber: 2g; Protein: 2g; Sugar: 3g

Italian-Inspired Rice and Peas

HIGH FIBER, GLUTEN-FREE, MEDIUM PROTEIN, VEGETARIAN

Serves 4 / Prep Time: 10 minutes / Cook Time: 35 minutes

This recipe is a renal take on the classic Italian recipe "risi e bisi." The traditional recipe calls for ham or pancetta. Omitting the meat reduces the dish's sodium and protein content. Using brown rice instead of white adds additional fiber and an earthy, nutty flavor. Feel free to try other grains, such as couscous or quinoa, in this recipe.

---

2 tablespoons extra-virgin olive oil

1 onion, chopped

1 cup brown rice

⅛ teaspoon salt

2½ cups water, divided

2 cups frozen baby peas

¼ teaspoon dried mint leaves

2 tablespoons grated
    Parmesan cheese

---

1. In a large saucepan, heat the olive oil over medium heat. Add the onion and cook for 2 to 3 minutes, stirring, until tender.

2. Add the rice and stir until the rice is coated with the oil. Sprinkle with the salt. Add 1 cup of water; cook for 5 to 10 minutes, stirring, until the water is absorbed.

3. Add another ½ cup of water; cook and stir until it's absorbed, another 5 minutes. Then add the remaining 1 cup of water, cover the pan, and simmer for about 20 minutes, stirring occasionally, until the rice is tender. Using this method will force the rice to omit some starch as it cooks, which makes the dish creamier.

4. Add the peas and mint to the pan. Cook for 3 to 5 minutes, stirring frequently, until the peas are hot and tender.

5. Sprinkle with the cheese and serve.

Make It Easier Tip: Use frozen precooked brown rice in place of the uncooked rice. Cook the onions in the olive oil, then add everything else except the cheese and cook over low heat until hot. Sprinkle with the cheese and serve.

Per Serving Calories: 317; Total fat: 10g; Saturated fat: 2g; Sodium: 207mg; Phosphorus: 237mg; Potassium: 312mg; Carbohydrates: 50g; Fiber: 5g; Protein: 9g; Sugar: 6g

Baked Jicama Fries

DIABETES-FRIENDLY, GLUTEN-FREE, HIGH FIBER, LOW PROTEIN, VEGETARIAN

Serves 4 / Prep Time: 20 minutes / Cook Time: 50 minutes

Native to Central America, jicama is a root vegetable that looks like a big round globe covered in brown skin. It's white and crunchy when you slice it, just like potatoes. When it's cut into sticks and baked with some seasonings, it's a great low-potassium, low-carb alternative to potato fries. Jicama is a good source of fiber and vitamin C.

1 pound jicama root
2 tablespoons butter
1 tablespoon extra-virgin olive oil
1 teaspoon chili powder
1 teaspoon paprika

¼ teaspoon salt
⅛ teaspoon freshly ground
   black pepper
2 tablespoons grated
   Parmesan cheese

1. Peel the jicama and cut into ½-inch slices. Cut the slices into strips, each about 4 inches long.

2. In a large saucepan, place the jicama strips and cover with water. Bring to a boil, then boil for 9 minutes. Drain the jicama well and transfer to a rimmed baking sheet. Pat the strips with a paper towel until they are dry, so the strips will crisp in the oven.

3. Preheat the oven to 400°F.

4. In a small saucepan, melt the butter with the olive oil. Drizzle over the jicama on the baking sheet. Sprinkle with the chili powder, paprika, salt, and pepper and toss to coat. Spread the strips into a single layer.

5. Bake the jicama fries for 40 to 45 minutes or until they are browned and crisp, turning once with a spatula halfway through the cooking time.

6. Sprinkle with the Parmesan cheese and serve.

Make It Easier Tip: You can buy precut jicama at many stores, including Trader Joe's. Make sure that you read the ingredients to confirm the package only contains jicama, not any preservatives or seasonings.

Per Serving Calories: 140; Total fat: 10g; Saturated fat: 5g; Sodium: 273mg; Phosphorus: 45mg; Potassium: 204mg; Carbohydrates: 11g; Fiber: 6g; Protein: 2g; Sugar: 2g

Double-Boiled Sweet Potatoes

GLUTEN-FREE, HIGH FIBER, LOW PROTEIN, VEGETARIAN

Serves 4 / Prep Time: 20 minutes / Cook Time: 25 minutes

Sweet potatoes are an excellent source of vitamin A, vitamin C, and fiber. Like most tubers, these spuds are also high in potassium, which can be problematic if you are following a low-potassium diet. It doesn't mean you have to omit them, however. The easy solution? Boil them twice! This double-boil method cuts the potassium content in potatoes by about half, and they still taste great.

2 large sweet potatoes, peeled and cut into 1-inch cubes	¼ cup half-and-half
2 tablespoons extra-virgin olive oil	1 tablespoon honey
2 tablespoons butter	¼ teaspoon salt
1 red onion, chopped	⅛ teaspoon freshly ground black pepper

1. In a large saucepan, fill the pot with water to about an inch above the potatoes. Add the sweet potato cubes and bring to a boil. Boil for 10 minutes.

2. Drain the sweet potatoes, discarding the water.

3. In the same saucepan, fill the pot to the same level again. Add the sweet potato cubes and bring to a boil. Boil for 10 to 15 minutes, or until the potatoes are tender.

4. Meanwhile, in a large skillet, heat the olive oil and butter. Add the red onion and cook for 3 to 5 minutes, stirring, until the onion is very tender.

5. Drain the sweet potatoes once more, discarding the water again. Add the sweet potatoes to the skillet along with the half-and-half, honey, salt, and pepper.

6. Mash the potatoes, using an immersion blender or a potato masher, until the desired consistency. Serve.

Make It Easier Tip: You can often find cubed sweet potatoes in the produce aisle at the supermarket. All you have to do is cut the cubes into smaller pieces, then proceed with the recipe.

Per Serving Calories: 246; Total fat: 14g; Saturated fat: 6g; Sodium: 235mg; Phosphorus: 62mg; Potassium: 201mg; Carbohydrates: 29g; Fiber: 3g; Protein: 2g; Sugar: 13g

Roasted Onion Dip

DIABETES-FRIENDLY, GLUTEN-FREE, LOW PROTEIN, VEGETARIAN

Makes about 1½ cups / Prep Time: 15 minutes / Cook Time: 35 minutes

Roasting onions completely changes their taste profile from harsh and pungent to tender and sweet. Onions should be a staple in any renal diet. They add tremendous flavor and contain heaps of health-promoting components, such as quercetin, a flavonoid linked to many health benefits including reduced inflammation and reduced blood pressure.

1 red onion, chopped
2 tablespoons extra-virgin olive oil
1 (8-ounce) package cream cheese, at room temperature

2 tablespoons mayonnaise (made with avocado oil or olive oil)
1 tablespoon freshly squeezed lemon juice
½ teaspoon dried thyme leaves

1. Preheat the oven to 400°F.

2. On a rimmed baking sheet, combine the onion and olive oil and toss to coat.

3. Roast for 30 to 35 minutes, stirring occasionally, until the onions are soft and golden brown. Don't let them burn. Transfer to a plate and set aside.

4. In a medium bowl, beat the cream cheese, mayonnaise, lemon juice, and thyme leaves. Stir in the onions.

5. You can serve the dip at this point or cover and refrigerate it up to 8 hours before serving.

Appliance Tip: You can roast onions in a slow cooker in larger quantities for bulk cooking or if you're throwing a party. Place 4 to 5 chopped onions and ¼ cup of olive oil in a 3-quart slow cooker. Cover and cook on low for 7 to 9 hours or until the onions are golden brown and tender. You can freeze the onions in ½-cup portions and add to soups, casseroles, side dishes, or stews.

Per Serving (3 tablespoons) Calories: 212; Total fat: 21g; Saturated fat: 9g; Sodium: 149mg; Phosphorus: 47mg; Potassium: 82mg; Carbohydrates: 4g; Fiber: 0g; Protein: 3g; Sugar: 2g

Roasted Garlic White Bean Dip

DIABETES-FRIENDLY, GLUTEN-FREE, HIGH FIBER, LOW PROTEIN, VEGAN

Makes 2 cups / Prep Time: 20 minutes / Cook Time: 1 hour

Roasting garlic and onion turns both vegetables into sweet and tender morsels that almost taste like candy. When pureed with some white beans, this dip makes for an excellent crudité appetizer or cracker topping. While beans are a high-potassium food, this recipe uses one can of cannellini beans to make six servings. If you plan to eat more than a serving at a time, be aware that you will also be taking in more potassium. Boiling the beans for about 10 minutes prior to preparing will reduce the potassium content by about 50 percent.

---

2 onions, cut into 8 wedges each

2 garlic heads, whole

¼ cup extra-virgin olive oil, divided

1 (15-ounce) can no-salt-added cannellini beans, drained and rinsed

2 tablespoons freshly squeezed lemon juice

1 teaspoon dried marjoram leaves

⅛ teaspoon salt

⅛ teaspoon freshly ground black pepper

---

1. Preheat the oven to 375°F.

2. On a rimmed baking sheet, place the onions.

3. Cut the top inch off each garlic head, just enough to expose the cloves, and discard the top. Place the garlic, with the exposed cloves facing up, on the baking sheet. Drizzle 1 tablespoon of olive oil directly into the garlic heads, then wrap each head in aluminum foil and place back on the baking sheet. Drizzle the onions with another 1 tablespoon of olive oil.

4. Roast the vegetables for 45 to 55 minutes, stirring the onions once during cooking, until the onions are golden brown and the garlic is brown and soft.

5. Remove the foil from the garlic and let the garlic and onions cool for 30 minutes.

6. In a blender or food processor, combine the cannellini beans, lemon juice, marjoram, salt, and pepper.

7. Add the onions. Remove the garlic cloves from the head by squeezing the head so the cloves pop out, and add to the blender. Blend or process the mixture, drizzling in the remaining 2 tablespoons of olive oil, until it is mostly smooth, with some texture.

8. Serve immediately or cover and chill for a few hours before serving.

Appliance Tip: You can roast the onions and garlic in a slow cooker. Just put the onion wedges in a 3-quart slow cooker. Separate the cloves from the garlic heads but don't peel them. Add 2 tablespoons of olive oil and 1 tablespoon of water to the slow cooker. Cover and cook on low for 7 to 9 hours, stirring a few times during the cooking time, until the vegetables are tender and brown. Slip the garlic cloves out of the skin and proceed with the recipe.

Per Serving (⅓ cup) Calories: 166; Total fat: 10g; Saturated fat: 1g; Sodium: 74mg; Phosphorus: 81mg; Potassium: 241mg; Carbohydrates: 17g; Fiber: 4g; Protein: 4g; Sugar: 2g

Green Goddess Dip

DIABETES-FRIENDLY, LOW PROTEIN, VEGETARIAN

Makes about 1½ cups / Prep Time: 15 minutes

Green Goddess is typically a salad dressing, made with mayonnaise, lemon juice, anchovies, and lots of fresh herbs. This version of the recipe is slightly different. Cream cheese is used instead of mayo and the anchovies are omitted, replaced by Worcestershire sauce. Serve it with fresh-cut raw vegetables such as carrots, celery, or cucumber slices.

1 (8-ounce) package cream cheese, at room temperature

3 tablespoons freshly squeezed lemon juice

2 teaspoons Worcestershire sauce

½ cup chopped flat-leaf parsley

¼ cup minced fresh chives

1. In a medium bowl, combine the cream cheese, lemon juice, and Worcestershire sauce and beat until smooth.

2. Stir in the parsley and chives. You can serve the dip immediately or cover and chill for 4 to 6 hours before serving.

Ingredient Tip: There are many other herbs you can add to this easy recipe, such as tarragon, basil, thyme, or sage. Fresh herbs are best because they tend to be more flavorful, but if you want to substitute dried herbs, use 1 teaspoon of dried herbs for every tablespoon of fresh.

Per Serving (3 tablespoons) Calories: 139; Total fat: 13g; Saturated fat: 8g; Sodium: 147mg; Phosphorus: 47mg; Potassium: 111mg; Carbohydrates: 4g; Fiber: 0g; Protein: 3g; Sugar: 2g

Crab and Carrot Dip

DIABETES-FRIENDLY, GLUTEN-FREE, MEDIUM PROTEIN

Makes about 1½ cups / Prep Time: 20 minutes

While crab dips are delicious, most contain little, if any, vegetables. This recipe changes that by incorporating scallions and carrots. This is an excellent recipe for entertaining and tastes even better when made ahead of time. You can use fresh or canned crab for this recipe, but avoid imitation crab meat because it's high in sodium and phosphorus.

1 cup mascarpone cheese

2 tablespoons freshly squeezed
   lemon juice

½ cup lump crab meat, drained

1 cup grated carrots

4 scallions, both green and white
   parts, chopped

1. In a medium bowl, beat the mascarpone and lemon juice until smooth.
2. Look over the crab, removing any bits of cartilage and discarding.
3. Stir the crab, carrots, and scallions into the mascarpone mixture. Serve immediately or cover and chill for 4 to 6 hours before serving.

Ingredient Tip: If using canned crab meat, look for a can that does not contain any phosphorus additives and choose the brand with the lowest sodium content per serving.

Per Serving (3 tablespoons) Calories: 194; Total fat: 18g; Saturated fat: 11g; Sodium: 146mg; Phosphorus: 89mg; Potassium: 184mg; Carbohydrates: 4g; Fiber: 1g; Protein: 5g; Sugar: 3g

Roasted Grape Crostini

HIGH FIBER, MEDIUM PROTEIN, VEGETARIAN

Serves 6 / Prep Time: 15 minutes / Cook Time: 25 minutes

Crostini is simply a combination of toasted bread and vegetables or fruit—sometimes with cheese. This unique version uses roasted grapes as a topping. Herbed cream cheese holds the grapes in place on the bread. Bread can be a high-sodium food. Slice the baguette about ¼-inch thick to limit the total sodium content.

1½ cups halved red grapes

3 tablespoons extra-virgin olive oil, divided

6 thin whole-wheat baguette slices

1 (8-ounce) package cream cheese, at room temperature

1 small shallot, minced

½ teaspoon dried thyme leaves

Pinch salt

Pinch freshly ground black pepper

1. Preheat the oven to 400°F.

2. Place the grapes on a jelly roll pan and drizzle with 1 tablespoon of olive oil and toss to coat.

3. Roast for 20 to 25 minutes or until the grapes are soft and lightly browned around the edges. Let cool for 20 minutes while you prepare the remaining ingredients.

4. Drizzle the bread with the remaining 2 tablespoons of olive oil and toast until golden brown.

5. In a small bowl, combine the cream cheese, shallot and thyme leaves and mix well.

6. Spread the cream cheese mixture on the bread and top with the grapes. Sprinkle with the salt and pepper and serve immediately.

Increase Protein Tip: To make this a high-protein recipe, reduce the cream cheese to 4 ounces and add 1 cup of plain nonfat Greek yogurt in step 4. The protein content will increase to 10g per serving.

Per Serving (1 crostini) Calories: 306; Total fat: 21g; Saturated fat: 9g; Sodium: 298mg; Phosphorus: 123mg; Potassium: 241mg; Carbohydrates: 24g; Fiber: 3g; Protein: 7g; Sugar: 9g

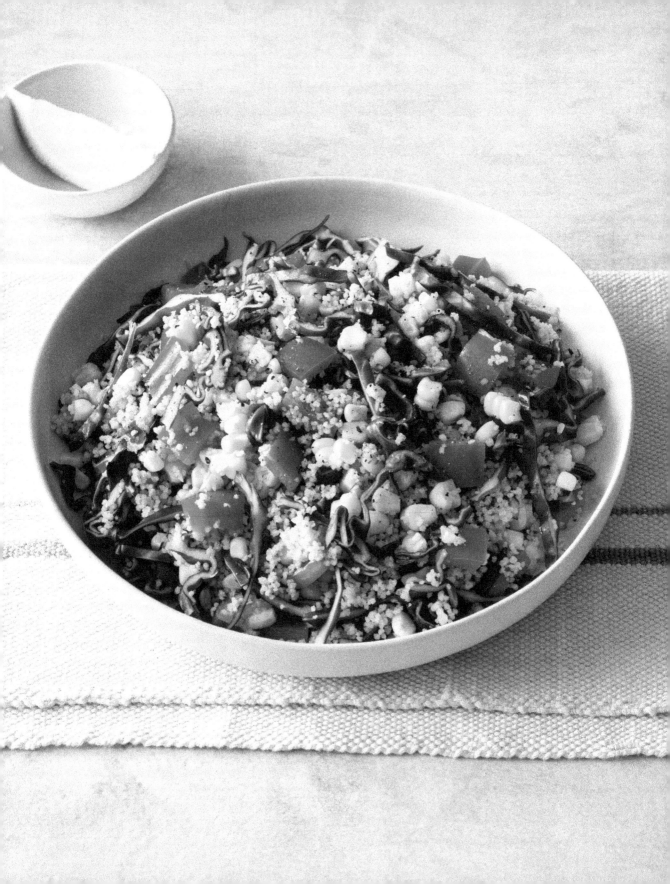

CHAPTER 4

Vegetarian and Vegan Entrées

⇐Cabbage Couscous Salad, page 54

Cabbage Couscous Salad

LOW PROTEIN, VEGAN

Serves 6 / Prep Time: 15 minutes / Cook Time: 10 minutes

Originating in North Africa, couscous is a dish of small, pearl-like balls made of crushed durum wheat, the same ingredient pasta is made from. It is rehydrated, not cooked, until it is fluffy and tender. It's delicious in a salad packed with vegetables and a light vinaigrette. If you can find the whole-wheat variety, use it, but if not, you'll still get plenty of fiber from the vegetables in this recipe.

¾ cup whole-wheat couscous

¾ cup water

4 tablespoons extra-virgin olive oil

2 tablespoons freshly squeezed
   lemon juice

⅛ teaspoon salt

⅛ teaspoon freshly ground
   black pepper

2 cups chopped red cabbage

1 cup frozen corn, thawed

1 red bell pepper, chopped

1. In a medium bowl, place the couscous. In a saucepan, bring the water to a boil and pour over the couscous. Cover the bowl and let stand for 10 minutes.

2. Meanwhile, in a serving bowl, combine the olive oil, lemon juice, salt, and pepper and whisk to combine.

3. Add the cabbage, corn, and bell pepper to the dressing and toss to coat.

4. When the couscous is tender, drain (if necessary), and add to the bowl. Toss gently to coat.

5. Serve immediately or cover and chill for 3 to 5 hours before serving.

Ingredient Tip: You can use any other vegetables you'd like in this fresh and colorful salad. Try sliced zucchini or yellow summer squash, cooked green beans, peas, or sliced celery.

Per Serving Calories: 196; Total fat: 10g; Saturated fat: 1g; Sodium: 57mg; Phosphorus: 66mg; Potassium: 223mg; Carbohydrates: 25g; Fiber: 4g; Protein: 4g; Sugar: 3g

Sweet and Sour Chickpeas

DIABETES-FRIENDLY, GLUTEN-FREE, HIGH FIBER, LOW PROTEIN, VEGAN

Serves 6 / Prep Time: 10 minutes / Cook Time: 12 minutes

Sweet and tangy ingredients add delicious flavor to chickpeas, which tend to be bland. Canned mixed tropical fruits add color and sweetness to this easy recipe. The sour is provided by lemon juice. Serve over hot cooked rice for a cheap and cheerful vegan dinner.

2 tablespoons extra-virgin olive oil

1 onion, chopped

1 (14-ounce) can tropical fruit in fruit juice, strained, reserving juice

2 tablespoons freshly squeezed lemon juice

2 tablespoons cornstarch

2 (15-ounce) cans no-salt-added chickpeas, drained and rinsed

1. In a large saucepan, heat the olive oil over medium heat. Cook the onion for 4 to 5 minutes, stirring frequently, until tender.

2. In a medium bowl, whisk together the fruit juice, lemon juice, and cornstarch.

3. When the onion is tender, add the chickpeas and cook for 3 to 4 minutes, stirring until hot.

4. Add the juice mixture and cook, stirring frequently, until the liquid is thickened, about 2 minutes.

5. Add the drained fruits to the saucepan and simmer for 1 to 2 minutes or until hot. Serve.

Ingredient Tip: You can find canned tropical fruit with no added sugar or other ingredients if you shop carefully. Native Forest Organic Tropical Fruit Salad is a good choice. Dole also makes a version with passion fruit juice that's delicious.

Per Serving Calories: 333; Total fat: 8g; Saturated fat: 1g; Sodium: 15mg; Phosphorus: 253mg; Potassium: 505mg; Carbohydrates: 54g; Fiber: 12g; Protein: 13g; Sugar: 17g

Cabbage-Stuffed Mushrooms

DIABETES-FRIENDLY, GLUTEN-FREE, LOW PROTEIN, VEGETARIAN

Serves 6 / Prep Time: 20 minutes / Cook Time: 25 minutes

You want a portobello mushroom for this recipe because of their large size. These sizeable mushrooms have a nice amount of space to hold the filling of your choosing. This recipe gets its flavor from tasty aromatic ingredients such as onion and ginger. Purchase pre-shredded cabbage to minimize prep time.

6 portobello mushrooms

3 tablespoons extra-virgin olive oil

1 onion, chopped

1 teaspoon minced peeled
   fresh ginger

2 cups shredded red cabbage

⅛ teaspoon salt

⅛ teaspoon freshly ground
   black pepper

3 tablespoons water

1 cup shredded Monterey
   Jack cheese

1. Rinse the mushrooms briefly and pat dry. Remove the stems and discard. Using a spoon, scrape out the dark gills on the underside of the mushroom cap. Set aside.

2. In a medium skillet, heat the olive oil over medium heat and cook the onion and ginger for 2 to 3 minutes, stirring, until fragrant.

3. Add the cabbage, salt, and pepper and sauté for 3 minutes, stirring frequently.

4. Add the water, cover, and steam the cabbage for 3 to 4 minutes, or until it is tender.

5. Remove the vegetables from the skillet and place in a medium bowl; let cool for 10 minutes, then stir in the cheese.

6. Preheat the oven to 400°F.

7. Place the caps on a baking sheet and divide the filling among the mushrooms. Bake for 15 to 17 minutes, or until the mushrooms are tender and the filling is light golden brown. Serve.

Per Serving Calories: 163; Total fat: 13g; Saturated fat: 5g; Sodium: 179mg; Phosphorus: 173mg; Potassium: 360mg; Carbohydrates: 7g; Fiber: 2g; Protein: 7g; Sugar: 3g

Ratatouille-Inspired Skewers

DIABETES-FRIENDLY, GLUTEN-FREE, LOW PROTEIN, VEGAN

Serves 4 / Prep Time: 20 minutes / Cook Time: 25 minutes

Ratatouille doesn't have to be made with a tomato sauce, as it is simply a dish consisting of a combination of vegetables. This version uses four different vegetables grilled on skewers. It is flavored with an herb blend to make a delicious and nutritious vegan main dish. The recipe yield allows four people to have three skewers each.

---

2 red onions, peeled and cut into 8 wedges

2 red bell peppers, cubed

1 eggplant, peeled and cut into cubes

12 large cherry tomatoes

⅓ cup extra-virgin olive oil, divided

1 teaspoon dried marjoram leaves, divided

⅛ teaspoon salt

⅛ teaspoon freshly ground black pepper

---

1. In a large bowl, place the onions, bell peppers, eggplant, and tomatoes and toss. Drizzle with ¼ cup of olive oil and sprinkle with ½ teaspoon of marjoram, the salt, and pepper. Let stand at room temperature for 30 minutes.

2. Prepare and preheat the grill to medium heat.

3. Thread the vegetables onto 12 metal skewers.

4. In a small bowl, combine the remaining 1½ tablespoons of olive oil and ½ teaspoon of marjoram.

5. Grill the vegetables for 12 to 17 minutes, turning several times while cooking and brushing with the reserved oil mixture, until the vegetables are tender. Serve over hot cooked brown rice or couscous.

Cooking Tip: You can roast these vegetables in the oven rather than grilling. Put the kebabs onto a rimmed baking sheet, preheat the oven to 400°F, and roast for 10 to 15 minutes or until the vegetables are tender. Brush the kebabs with the reserved oil mixture twice during the cooking time.

Per Serving Calories: 80; Total fat: 6g; Saturated fat: 1g; Sodium: 29mg; Phosphorus: 26mg; Potassium: 219mg; Carbohydrates: 6g; Fiber: 2g; Protein: 1g; Sugar: 4g

Curried Veggie Stir-Fry

DIABETES-FRIENDLY, GLUTEN-FREE, HIGH FIBER, LOW PROTEIN, VEGAN

Serves 6 / Prep Time: 20 minutes / Cook Time: 10 minutes

A stir-fry is one of the quickest ways to prepare a meal but be forewarned: all the ingredients must be prepared before you start cooking. You can make this satisfying recipe as mild or as spicy as you like depending on the type of curry paste you choose. Green is the hottest, red is medium hot, and yellow is the mildest. This stir-fry tastes great on its own or paired with rice or noodles.

2 tablespoons extra-virgin olive oil

1 onion, chopped

4 garlic cloves, minced

4 cups frozen stir-fry vegetables

1 cup canned unsweetened full-fat coconut milk

1 cup water

2 tablespoons green curry paste

1. In a wok or nonstick skillet, heat the olive oil over medium-high heat. Stir-fry the onion and garlic for 2 to 3 minutes, until fragrant.

2. Add the frozen stir-fry vegetables and continue to cook for 3 to 4 minutes longer, or until the vegetables are hot.

3. Meanwhile, in a small bowl, combine coconut milk, water, and curry paste. Stir until the paste dissolves.

4. Add the broth mixture to the wok and cook for another 2 to 3 minutes, or until the sauce has reduced slightly and all the vegetables are crisp-tender. Serve over couscous or hot cooked rice.

Ingredient Tip: When you buy frozen stir-fry vegetables, make sure you purchase a variety that doesn't include seasonings or sauce, which would increase the sodium content. You could also use separate veggies; try a combination of broccoli with carrots or asparagus with zucchini.

Per Serving Calories: 293; Total fat: 18g; Saturated fat: 10g; Sodium: 247mg; Phosphorus: 138mg; Potassium: 531mg; Carbohydrates: 28g; Fiber: 7g; Protein: 7g; Sugar: 4g

Spicy Corn and Rice Burritos

GLUTEN-FREE, LOW PROTEIN, VEGETARIAN

Serves 4 / Prep Time: 10 minutes / Cook Time: 20 minutes

Burritos are one of the world's most popular foods—and for good reason. They taste great and can be enjoyed for breakfast, lunch, and dinner. This vegetarian recipe is full of flavor and easy to make. You can serve the burritos without frying, or go ahead and fry them in olive oil for a crispy, yet healthy, treat.

3 tablespoons extra-virgin olive oil, divided

1 (10-ounce) package frozen cooked brown rice

1½ cups frozen yellow corn

1 tablespoon chili powder

1 cup shredded pepper jack cheese

4 large or 6 small corn tortillas

1. In a medium skillet, heat 2 tablespoons of olive oil over medium heat. Add the rice, corn, and chili powder and cook for 4 to 6 minutes, or until the ingredients are hot.

2. Transfer the ingredients from the pan into a medium bowl. Let cool for 15 minutes.

3. Stir the cheese into the rice mixture.

4. Heat the tortillas as directed on the package to make them pliable. Fill the corn tortillas with the rice mixture, then roll them up.

5. At this point, you can serve them as is, or you can fry them first. Heat the remaining tablespoon of olive oil in a large skillet. Fry the burritos, seam-side down at first, turning once, until they are brown and crisp, about 4 to 6 minutes per side, then serve.

Diabetes Tip: To make this recipe diabetes-friendly substitute frozen cauliflower rice for the brown rice. This will also make the recipe high fiber.

Per Serving Calories: 386; Total fat: 21g; Saturated fat: 7g; Sodium: 510mg; Phosphorus: 304mg; Potassium: 282mg; Carbohydrates: 41g; Fiber: 4g; Protein: 11g; Sugar: 2g

Red Beans and Rice

DIABETES-FRIENDLY, GLUTEN-FREE, HIGH FIBER, LOW PROTEIN, VEGAN

Serves 4 / Prep Time: 10 minutes / Cook Time: 1 hour

Legumes, including red beans, are an excellent source of fiber. A traditional Creole red beans and rice recipe uses smoked andouille sausage. Processed meat, such as sausage, should be avoided on a renal diet because it's high in sodium and often contains phosphorus additives. This vegan recipe omits this ingredient, relying instead on the flavor of chili powder and vegetables.

2¾ cups low-sodium vegetable broth, divided

1 cup brown rice

1 (15-ounce) can no-salt-added kidney beans, drained and rinsed, reserving 2 tablespoons packing liquid

3 tablespoons extra-virgin olive oil

2 cups frozen pepper and onion blend

1 tablespoon chili powder

⅛ teaspoon salt

⅛ teaspoon freshly ground black pepper

1. In a large saucepan, combine 2¼ cups of vegetable stock and the brown rice. Bring to a boil over high heat, then reduce the heat to low, partially cover the pan, and simmer for 30 to 35 minutes, or until the rice is tender. Drain if necessary and set aside.

2. In a medium saucepan, place the beans, cover with water, and bring to a boil. Simmer for 10 minutes, then drain off the cooking liquid.

3. Meanwhile, in a large skillet, heat the olive oil over medium heat. Add the frozen vegetables and cook for 5 to 6 minutes, stirring, until thawed.

4. Add the beans and the reserved packing liquid from the can, along with the remaining ½ cup of vegetable stock, to the skillet with the vegetables. Sprinkle with the chili powder, salt, and pepper.

5. Reduce the heat to low and simmer for 5 to 10 minutes, stirring occasionally, until the vegetables are hot and tender.

6. When the vegetables and rice are done cooking, place them in separate serving bowls. Serve the beans topped with a scoop of the rice.

Make It Easier Tip: You can buy frozen brown rice and thaw it instead of cooking it from scratch to save about 30 minutes. Omit most of the vegetable stock; use only the ½ cup added to the vegetables.

Increase Protein Tip: To make this a medium-protein recipe, accompany each serving with 1 egg fried in olive oil. The protein content will increase to 20g per serving.

Per Serving Calories: 432; Total fat: 13g; Saturated fat: 2g; Sodium: 232 mg; Phosphorus: 304mg; Potassium: 599mg; Carbohydrates: 67g; Fiber: 9g; Protein: 13g; Sugar: 8g

Chilaquiles

DIABETES-FRIENDLY, GLUTEN-FREE, MEDIUM PROTEIN, VEGETARIAN

Serves 4 / Prep Time: 20 minutes / Cook Time: 20 minutes

Chilaquiles combine crisp tortilla strips, a sauce, and cooked eggs. It's usually served for breakfast but also makes an excellent quick lunch or dinner. Tomatillos are used instead of red enchilada sauce. These little green "tomatoes" are spicy and fresh tasting. For more protein, use 8 whole eggs, increasing the protein to 25 grams per serving.

3 (8-inch) corn tortillas, cut into strips

2 tablespoons extra-virgin olive oil

12 tomatillos, papery covering removed, chopped

3 tablespoons freshly squeezed lime juice

⅛ teaspoon salt

⅛ teaspoon freshly ground black pepper

4 large egg whites

2 large eggs

2 tablespoons water

1 cup shredded pepper jack cheese

1. In a dry nonstick skillet, toast the tortilla strips over medium heat until they are crisp, tossing the pan and stirring occasionally. This should take 4 to 6 minutes. Remove the strips from the pan and set aside.

2. In the same skillet, heat the olive oil over medium heat and add the tomatillos, lime juice, salt, and pepper. Cook for 8 to 10 minutes, stirring frequently, until the tomatillos start to break down and form a sauce. Transfer the sauce to a bowl and set aside.

3. In a small bowl, beat the egg whites, eggs, and water and add to the skillet. Cook the eggs for 3 to 4 minutes, stirring occasionally, until they are set and cooked to 160°F.

4. Preheat the oven to 400°F.

5. Toss the tortilla strips in the tomatillo sauce and place in a casserole dish. Top with the scrambled eggs and cheese.

6. Bake for 10 to 15 minutes, or until the cheese starts to brown. Serve.

Per Serving Calories: 312; Total fat: 20g; Saturated fat: 8g; Sodium: 345mg; Phosphorus: 280mg; Potassium: 453mg; Carbohydrates: 19g; Fiber: 3g; Protein: 15g; Sugar: 5g

Creamy Mushroom Pasta

HIGH FIBER, LOW PROTEIN, VEGETARIAN

Serves 6 / Prep Time: 10 minutes / Cook Time: 20 minutes

Even everyday button mushrooms are flavorful when cooked with butter and garlic. This easy recipe can be made in under 20 minutes and it's a great comforting weeknight standby. Save time on prepping by purchasing pre-peeled garlic.

12 ounces whole-grain
   fettuccine pasta
3 tablespoons extra-virgin olive oil
1 (8-ounce) package button
   mushrooms, sliced

3 garlic cloves, sliced
1 cup heavy cream
Pinch salt
Freshly ground black pepper

1. Bring a large pot of water to a boil. Add the pasta and cook for 9 to 10 minutes, until al dente. Drain, reserving about ⅓ cup of the pasta water, and set aside.

2. Meanwhile, in a large heavy saucepan, heat the olive oil on medium-high heat. Add the mushrooms in a single layer. Cook for 3 minutes or until the mushrooms are golden brown on one side. Carefully turn the mushrooms and cook for another 2 minutes.

3. Reduce the heat to medium and add the garlic. Sauté, stirring, for 2 minutes longer, until the garlic is fragrant.

4. Add the cream to the skillet with the mushrooms and season with salt and pepper. Simmer for 3 minutes or until the mixture starts to thicken.

5. Add the drained pasta to the pan and coat using tongs. Add the reserved pasta water if necessary, to loosen the sauce. Serve.

Increase Protein Tip: To make this a medium-protein recipe, replace the whole-wheat pasta with chickpea or lentil pasta. The protein content will increase to 18g per serving. If you are following a low-potassium diet, opt for chickpea pasta as other legume pastas are higher in potassium.

Per Serving Calories: 405; Total fat: 23g; Saturated fat: 10g; Sodium: 42mg; Phosphorus: 252mg; Potassium: 410mg; Carbohydrates: 44g; Fiber: 6g; Protein: 10g; Sugar: 3g

Crustless Cabbage Quiche

DIABETES-FRIENDLY, GLUTEN-FREE, LOW PROTEIN, VEGETARIAN

Serves 6 / Prep Time: 10 minutes / Cook Time: 40 minutes

You won't miss the crust in this easy, gluten-free recipe. Purchasing a coleslaw blend will save you the task of shredding cabbage and carrots. The Swiss cheese, half-and-half, and dill combine beautifully in this rich and flavorful vegetarian recipe. With only one egg per serving, this recipe is also low in protein.

Olive oil cooking spray

2 tablespoons extra-virgin olive oil

3 cups coleslaw blend with carrots

3 large eggs, beaten

3 large egg whites, beaten

½ cup half-and-half

1 teaspoon dried dill weed

⅛ teaspoon salt

⅛ teaspoon freshly ground black pepper

1 cup grated Swiss cheese

1. Preheat the oven to 350°F. Spray a 9-inch pie plate with cooking spray and set aside.

2. In a large skillet, heat the olive oil over medium heat. Add the coleslaw mix and cook for 4 to 6 minutes, stirring, until the cabbage is tender. Transfer the vegetables from the pan to a medium bowl to cool.

3. Meanwhile, in another medium bowl, combine the eggs and egg whites, half-and-half, dill, salt, and pepper and beat to combine.

4. Stir the cabbage mixture into the egg mixture and pour into the prepared pie plate.

5. Sprinkle with the cheese.

6. Bake for 30 to 35 minutes, or until the mixture is puffed, set, and light golden brown. Let stand for 5 minutes, then slice to serve.

Ingredient Tip: Separating egg whites from egg yolks can be a nuisance. To save time, purchase liquid egg whites in a carton and simply pour the amount that is needed in the recipe.

Per Serving Calories: 203; Total fat: 16g; Saturated fat: 6g; Sodium: 321mg; Phosphorus: 169mg; Potassium: 155mg; Carbohydrates: 5g; Fiber: 1g; Protein: 11g; Sugar: 4g

Roasted Veggie Sandwiches

LOW PROTEIN, VEGAN

Serves 6 / Prep Time: 20 minutes / Cook Time: 35 minutes

When roasted in olive oil, vegetables develop a wonderful texture, creating the perfect filling for pita bread. Balsamic vinegar is the winning ingredient in this recipe. Purchase a good-quality balsamic vinegar and enjoy the delicious sweet and smoky flavor it brings to this dish.

---

3 bell peppers, assorted
  colors, sliced
1 cup sliced yellow summer squash
1 red onion, sliced
2 tablespoons extra-virgin olive oil
2 tablespoons balsamic vinegar

⅛ teaspoon salt
⅛ teaspoon freshly ground
  black pepper
3 large whole-wheat pita
  breads, halved

---

1. Preheat the oven to 400°F. Line a rimmed baking sheet with parchment paper.
2. Spread the bell peppers, squash, and onion on the prepared baking sheet. Sprinkle with the olive oil, vinegar, salt, and pepper.
3. Roast for 30 to 40 minutes, turning the vegetables with a spatula once during cooking, until they are tender and light golden brown.
4. Pile the vegetables into the pita breads and serve.

Ingredient Tip: Pita breads are puffed rounds that have a natural pocket in the center that holds a filling. To prepare them, cut in half crosswise and gently separate the two halves, cutting the pocket if necessary. You can find pita breads in most supermarkets.

Per Serving Calories: 182; Total fat: 5g; Saturated fat: 1g; Sodium: 234mg; Phosphorus: 106mg; Potassium: 289mg; Carbohydrates: 31g; Fiber: 4g; Protein: 5g; Sugar: 6g

Roasted Peach Open-Face Sandwich

LOW PROTEIN, VEGETARIAN

Serves 4 / Prep Time: 5 minutes / Cook Time: 15 minutes

Instead of relying on typical sandwich ingredients, such as processed meat and cheese, why not try fruit? This recipe uses roasted peaches that contribute tangy and sweet flavor. This sandwich is delicious served for lunch or dinner.

2 fresh peaches, peeled and sliced

1 tablespoon extra-virgin olive oil

1 tablespoon freshly squeezed lemon juice

⅛ teaspoon salt

⅛ teaspoon freshly ground black pepper

4 ounces cream cheese, at room temperature

2 teaspoons fresh thyme leaves

4 whole-wheat sourdough bread slices

1. Preheat the oven to 400°F.

2. Arrange the peaches on a rimmed baking sheet. Brush them with the olive oil on both sides.

3. Roast the peaches for 10 to 15 minutes, until they are light golden brown around the edges. Sprinkle with the lemon juice, salt, and pepper.

4. In a small bowl, combine the cream cheese and thyme and mix well.

5. Toast the bread and spread with the cream cheese mixture. Top with the peaches and serve.

Per Serving Calories: 250; Total fat: 13g; Saturated fat: 6g; Sodium: 376mg; Phosphorus: 163mg; Potassium: 260mg; Carbohydrates: 28g; Fiber: 3g; Protein: 6g; Sugar: 8g

Pasta Fagioli

HIGH FIBER, LOW PROTEIN, VEGETARIAN

Serves 6 / Prep Time: 25 minutes / Cook Time: 25 minutes

Pasta fagioli is an Italian soup recipe that combines pasta and beans. It's rich, comforting, and easy to make. While most pasta fagioli recipes use tomatoes, this recipe omits them to control the total potassium content. A portion of vegetables and beans are pureed together to give the soup body and color.

1 (15-ounce) can low-sodium great northern beans, drained and rinsed, divided

2 cups frozen peppers and onions, thawed, divided

5 cups low-sodium vegetable broth

⅛ teaspoon salt

⅛ teaspoon freshly ground black pepper

1 cup whole-grain orecchiette pasta

2 tablespoons extra-virgin olive oil

⅓ cup grated Parmesan cheese

1. In a large saucepan, place the beans and cover with water. Bring to a boil over high heat and boil for 10 minutes. Drain the beans.

2. In a food processor or blender, combine ⅓ cup of beans and ⅓ cup of thawed peppers and onions. Process until smooth.

3. In the same saucepan, combine the pureed mixture, the remaining 1⅔ cups of peppers and onions, the remaining beans, the broth, and the salt and pepper and bring to a simmer.

4. Add the pasta to the saucepan and stir. Bring to a boil, reduce the heat to low, and simmer for 8 to 10 minutes, or until the pasta is tender.

5. Serve drizzled with olive oil and topped with Parmesan cheese.

Appliance Tip: If you don't have a blender or food processor, you can use a potato masher.

Diabetes Tip: To make this recipe diabetes-friendly, reduce or completely eliminate the amount of pasta in the recipe. Feel free to replace the pasta with extra vegetables, such as chopped mushrooms or carrots.

Per Serving Calories: 245; Total fat: 7g; Saturated fat: 2g; Sodium: 269mg; Phosphorus: 188mg; Potassium: 592mg; Carbohydrates: 36g; Fiber: 7g; Protein: 12g; Sugar: 4g

Spinach Alfredo Lasagna Rolls

DIABETES-FRIENDLY, HIGH FIBER, LOW PROTEIN, VEGETARIAN

Serves 4 / Prep Time: 25 minutes / Cook Time: 50 minutes

Lasagna has to be the ultimate comfort food, but it uses a lot of tomatoes and a lot of pasta. This version uses a simple white sauce that is made with cream cheese and reserved pasta cooking water, which has some starch to make the sauce smooth.

---

4 whole-grain lasagna noodles

2 tablespoons extra-virgin olive oil

1 large onion, chopped

2 cups frozen whole-leaf spinach, thawed (measure while frozen)

1 (8-ounce) package cream cheese, at room temperature, divided

⅓ cup shredded Parmesan cheese

---

1. Bring a large pot of water to a boil over high heat and add the lasagna noodles. Simmer for 8 to 9 minutes or until the pasta is almost al dente but still has a thin white line in the center. Drain, reserving ¼ cup of the pasta water, and set aside.

2. Meanwhile, in a saucepan, heat the olive oil over medium heat. Add the onions and cook for 6 to 8 minutes, stirring, until the onions are tender and starting to turn brown.

3. While the onions are cooking, drain the spinach and put the leaves into some paper towels. Squeeze well to remove most of the water from the spinach.

4. Add the spinach to the onions, stir, and turn off the heat. Add 6 ounces of cream cheese to the vegetables and stir until combined. Set aside.

5. In a small saucepan, combine the remaining 2 ounces of cream cheese with the reserved pasta water. Heat over low heat, stirring often with a wire whisk, until smooth.

6. In a 9-inch baking dish, place 2 tablespoons of the cream cheese sauce.

7. On a work surface, place the lasagna noodles. Divide the spinach mixture among them and roll them up.

8. Place the rolls, seam-side down, on the sauce in the casserole. Top with the remaining sauce.

9. Sprinkle the lasagna rolls with the Parmesan cheese. Bake for 25 to 35 minutes, or until the lasagna is bubbling and the top starts to brown.

Make It Easier Tip: To reduce the prep time, you can purchase no-boil lasagna noodles. You won't have any reserved pasta water to use for step 7, so just use plain water instead.

Per Serving Calories: 388; Total fat: 24g; Saturated fat: 7g; Sodium: 411mg; Phosphorus: 119mg; Potassium: 378mg; Carbohydrates: 34g; Fiber: 9g; Protein: 13g; Sugar: 5g

Pepper Jack and Rice Stuffed Peppers

GLUTEN-FREE, HIGH FIBER, LOW PROTEIN, VEGETARIAN

Serves 4 / Prep Time: 20 minutes / Cook Time: 65 minutes

Stuffed peppers are a classic recipe. The filling usually includes some type of meat, but this vegetarian version is just as delicious. Using brown rice boosts the dish's fiber content. Alternatively, you could use wild rice, a darker rice with a rich and nutty flavor.

6 red bell peppers

2 tablespoons extra-virgin olive oil

1 onion, chopped

½ teaspoon Italian seasoning

⅛ teaspoon salt

⅛ teaspoon freshly ground black pepper

2 cups cooked brown rice

⅔ cup shredded pepper jack cheese

1. Cut the top inch off of 4 peppers. Then use a knife and your fingers to remove the seeds and light-colored membranes from the inside of the peppers and set aside. Be careful so you don't split the peppers or cut a hole in the bottom.

2. Seed and chop the remaining 2 bell peppers.

3. Preheat the oven to 375°F.

4. In a large saucepan, heat the olive oil over medium heat. Add the onion and cook for about 3 minutes, stirring, until crisp-tender.

5. Add the chopped bell peppers. Sprinkle with the Italian seasoning, salt, and pepper. Cook and stir for 3 to 5 minutes or until crisp tender. Stir in the brown rice and remove from the heat.

6. Stir the cheese into the vegetable mixture.

7. Place the bell peppers into a casserole dish so they fit snugly. Fill each pepper with the vegetable mixture.

8. Pour ½ cup of water into the casserole dish, around the bell peppers. Cover the dish with aluminum foil.

9. Bake for 35 minutes, then remove the foil. Bake for another 20 to 25 minutes or until the peppers are tender and the filling is brown on top.

Appliance Tip: You can cook this recipe in the slow cooker. Choose a smaller slow cooker so the peppers fit snugly. Prepare as directed but add only ¼ cup of water to the bottom of the slow cooker. Cover and cook on high for 3 hours or on low for 6 hours until the peppers are tender.

Per Serving Calories: 316; Total fat: 14g; Saturated fat: 5g; Sodium: 202mg; Phosphorus: 249mg; Potassium: 580mg; Carbohydrates: 40g; Fiber: 6g; Protein: 9g; Sugar: 9g

Creamy Veggie Casserole

DIABETES-FRIENDLY, LOW PROTEIN, VEGAN

Serves 4 / Prep Time: 25 minutes / Cook Time: 35 minutes

This is a warm and comforting dish, a perfect dinner for a cold winter night. The crust for this recipe is made from crushed rice cereal, which is much lower in sodium compared to conventional bread crumbs. It also happens to be gluten-free. California blend vegetables refer to the combination of broccoli, cauliflower, and carrots.

⅓ cup extra-virgin olive oil, divided

1 onion, chopped

2 tablespoons flour

3 cups low-sodium vegetable broth

3 cups frozen California blend vegetables

1 cup crushed crisp rice cereal

1. Preheat the oven to 375°F.
2. In a large saucepan, heat 2 tablespoons of olive oil over medium heat. Add the onion and cook for 3 to 4 minutes, stirring, until the onion is tender.
3. Add the flour and stir for 2 minutes.
4. Add the broth to the saucepan, stirring for 3 to 4 minutes, or until the sauce starts to thicken.
5. Add the vegetables to the saucepan. Bring to a simmer and cook for 6 to 8 minutes, or until the vegetables are hot and tender.
6. When the vegetables are done, pour the mixture into a 3-quart casserole dish.
7. Sprinkle the vegetables with the crushed cereal.
8. Bake for 20 to 25 minutes or until the cereal is golden brown and the filling is bubbling. Let cool for 5 minutes and serve.

Ingredient Tip: Adding 1 cup of your favorite shredded cheese will give this recipe a little something extra.

Per Serving Calories: 234; Total fat: 18g; Saturated fat: 3g; Sodium: 139mg; Phosphorus: 21mg; Potassium: 210mg; Carbohydrates: 16g; Fiber: 3g; Protein: 3g; Sugar: 5g

Pad Thai

DIABETES-FRIENDLY, HIGH FIBER, MEDIUM PROTEIN, VEGAN

Serves 4 / Prep Time: 20 minutes / Cook Time: 20 minutes

Pad Thai is made of thin pasta strands that are cooked and stir-fried with veggies and a spicy peanut sauce. Restaurant pad Thai contains excessive amounts of sodium. This recipe contains considerably less sodium and everything is stir-fried in heart-healthy olive oil. This recipe is ideal for a quick weeknight dinner.

8 ounces whole-grain spaghetti or capellini

3 tablespoons extra-virgin olive oil

2 cups frozen stir-fry vegetables

⅓ cup peanut butter

2 tablespoons low-sodium soy sauce

¼ teaspoon freshly ground black pepper

1 lime, juiced and zested

1. Bring a large pot of water to a boil. Add the pasta and boil until al dente. Remove ⅓ cup of the pasta water and set aside. Drain the pasta and also set aside.

2. In a large saucepan, heat the olive oil over medium-high heat. Add the vegetables, reduce the heat to medium, and stir-fry for 3 to 6 minutes, or until they are thawed.

3. Meanwhile, in a small bowl, combine the peanut butter, reserved pasta water, soy sauce, and pepper and beat well.

4. When the vegetables are thawed, add the drained pasta and stir-fry for 2 minutes or until hot.

5. Add the peanut butter sauce. Stir-fry until the sauce has thickened and coats the pasta.

6. Stir in the lime juice and zest and serve.

Ingredient Tip: Zest the limes before you squeeze them for juice or zesting will be very difficult. Use a zester or the tiniest holes on your box grater to zest. Avoid grating the white pith, as it is bitter.

Per Serving Calories: 453; Total fat: 22g; Saturated fat: 4g; Sodium: 397mg; Phosphorus: 267mg; Potassium: 417mg; Carbohydrates: 56g; Fiber: 8g; Protein: 15g; Sugar: 5g

Vegetable Green Curry

DIABETES-FRIENDLY, GLUTEN-FREE, HIGH FIBER, LOW PROTEIN, VEGETARIAN

Serves 6 / Prep Time: 20 minutes / Cook Time: 20 minutes

If curry dishes are not part of your usual repertoire, it may be time to add them to the menu. Many people are put off by the word "curry," and incorrectly assume that the dish will be too spicy for their palate. While curry dishes all contain spices, this does not necessarily mean the dish will be overly spicy. Green curry paste adds great flavor and enhances the green color of the other vegetables used in this dish. You can serve it as-is, or pour it over cooked rice.

2 tablespoons extra-virgin olive oil

1 head broccoli, cut into florets

1 bunch asparagus, cut into 2-inch lengths

3 tablespoons water

2 tablespoons green curry paste

1 medium eggplant

⅛ teaspoon salt

⅛ teaspoon freshly ground black pepper

⅔ cup plain whole-milk yogurt

1. In a large saucepan, heat the olive oil over medium heat. Add the broccoli and stir-fry for 5 minutes. Add the asparagus and stir-fry for another 3 minutes.

2. Meanwhile, in a small bowl, combine the water with the green curry paste.

3. Add the eggplant, curry-water mixture, salt, and pepper. Stir-fry for another 3 to 5 minutes or until vegetables are all tender.

4. Add the yogurt. Heat through but avoid simmering. Serve.

Ingredient Tip: For a spicier curry, you could add 2 teaspoons of curry powder, or use yellow or red curry paste instead of the green version.

Per Serving Calories: 113; Total fat: 6g; Saturated fat: 1g; Sodium: 174mg; Phosphorus: 117mg; Potassium: 569mg; Carbohydrates: 13g; Fiber: 6g; Protein: 5g; Sugar: 7g

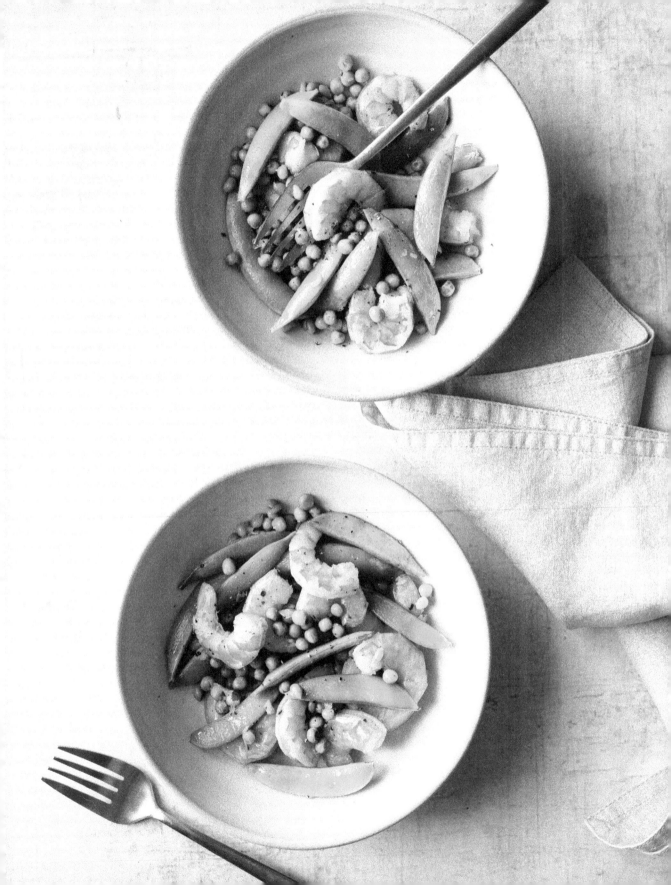

CHAPTER 5

Fish, Poultry, and Meat

⇦Ginger Shrimp with Snow Peas, page 82

Corn and Shrimp Quiche

DIABETES-FRIENDLY, GLUTEN-FREE, MEDIUM PROTEIN

Serves 6 / Prep Time: 15 minutes / Cook Time: 50 minutes

Don't you love how many different dishes you can make with eggs? A quiche is a versatile and healthy meal idea perfect for breakfast, lunch, or even dinner. Leaving out the crust makes it healthier and simpler to make. The shrimp adds wonderful texture and flavor. This recipe calls for small shrimp, which number about 50 in a pound.

1 cup small cooked shrimp

1½ cups frozen corn, thawed and drained

¾ cup shredded sharp Colby cheese

5 large eggs, beaten

1 cup unsweetened almond milk

Pinch salt

⅛ teaspoon freshly ground black pepper

1. Preheat the oven to 350°F. Spray a 9-inch pie pan with nonstick baking spray.

2. In the prepared pan, combine the shrimp and corn. Sprinkle the cheese over top.

3. In a medium bowl, beat the eggs, almond milk, salt, and pepper. Gently pour into the pan.

4. Bake for 45 to 55 minutes or until the quiche is puffed, set to the touch, and light golden brown on top. Let stand for 10 minutes before cutting into wedges to serve.

Ingredient Tip: Shrimp are measured according to the number per pound. So bigger shrimp have a lower number per pound. For this recipe, small shrimp should be about 50 per pound. Medium shrimp are usually 36 to 40 per pound. You can cut larger shrimp into small pieces instead of buying small shrimp if you'd like.

Per Serving (1 slice) Calories: 198; Total fat: 10g; Saturated fat: 4g; Sodium: 238mg; Phosphorus: 260mg; Potassium: 261mg; Carbohydrates: 9g; Fiber: 1g; Protein: 20g; Sugar: 2g

Ginger-Orange Tuna Pasta Salad

Serves 6 / Prep Time: 20 minutes / Cook Time: 9 minutes, plus 2 hours to chill

This pasta salad is a delicious dish to serve for large groups and is easy to prepare. You can have the recipe prepped long before people arrive so that you can focus on your guests! Always look for light tuna; other types of tuna are high in mercury, a toxin that has been linked to renal damage. Light tuna has the lowest mercury content.

3 cups whole-wheat ziti pasta

1 large navel orange, zested and juiced

¼ cup extra-virgin olive oil

2 tablespoons yellow prepared mustard

¼ teaspoon ground ginger

Pinch salt

1 large navel orange, peeled and segmented

1 (6-ounce) can light low-sodium tuna, drained

1. Bring a large pot of water to a boil. Add the pasta and cook according to package directions, until the pasta is al dente. Drain and set aside.

2. In a large bowl, whisk the orange juice and zest, olive oil, mustard, ginger, and salt until combined. Add the orange segments and tuna and stir to coat.

3. When the pasta is done, drain and add to the bowl with the dressing and other ingredients. Toss to coat.

4. Cover and chill the salad for 2 to 3 hours, stirring once.

Increase Protein Tip: To make this a medium-protein recipe, add one more can of drained tuna. The protein content will increase to 19g per serving.

Per Serving Calories: 305; Total fat: 11g; Saturated fat: 2g; Sodium: 105mg; Phosphorus: 218mg; Potassium: 379mg; Carbohydrates: 43g; Fiber: 6g; Protein: 13g; Sugar: 7g

Pineapple-Soy Salmon Stir-Fry

DIABETES-FRIENDLY, MEDIUM PROTEIN

Serves 4 / Prep Time: 15 minutes / Cook Time: 15 minutes

Stir-fry meals are a wonderful way to cook big amounts of healthy vegetables with small amounts of animal protein. This colorful and flavorful stir-fry uses just 12 ounces of salmon fillets to serve four people, yet it's very satisfying and filling. Before cooking a stir-fry, make sure to have all the ingredients prepped and ready to go, as the cooking process is very quick.

1 (8-ounce) can crushed pineapple, strained, reserving juice
2 tablespoons low-sodium soy sauce
1 tablespoon cornstarch
⅛ teaspoon freshly ground black pepper

2 tablespoons extra-virgin olive oil
2 (6-ounce) salmon fillets without skin, cubed
1 (16-ounce) bag frozen stir-fry vegetables

1. In a small bowl, whisk the reserved pineapple juice, soy sauce, cornstarch, and pepper and set aside.

2. In a large wok or skillet, heat the olive oil. Add the salmon cubes and stir-fry for 3 to 4 minutes, or until the salmon flakes with a fork. Using a slotted spoon, transfer the salmon to a plate and set aside.

3. Add the frozen vegetables to the wok and stir-fry for another 3 to 4 minutes, or until the vegetables are hot and tender.

4. Return the salmon to the wok and add the pineapple.

5. Whisk the sauce again and add to the wok; stir-fry for 3 to 4 minutes or until the sauce bubbles and has thickened. Serve.

Ingredient Tip: You can make this recipe with just about any protein, such as cubed boneless skinless chicken breasts, cod or sole, or peeled and deveined shrimp. To make this recipe gluten-free, use low-sodium tamari instead of soy sauce.

Per Serving Calories: 280; Total fat: 13g; Saturated fat: 2g; Sodium: 361mg; Phosphorus: 271mg; Potassium: 599mg; Carbohydrates: 21g; Fiber: 3g; Protein: 22g; Sugar: 11g

Fish Taco Filling

Serves 4 / Prep Time: 15 minutes / Cook Time: 10 minutes

Tacos are so versatile, and all you need is your imagination to create your own self-styled taco. There are endless possibilities for fun fillings so you never get bored. In this easily prepared recipe, sautéed sole is paired with the healthy crunch of cabbage coleslaw. The drizzle of lime juice adds a refreshing zing to this light dish. Serve this in corn tortillas to make tacos or spoon over hot cooked rice.

2 tablespoons extra-virgin olive oil

2 shallots, minced

3 (6-ounce) sole fillets, cut into strips

2 teaspoons chili powder

1 lime, zested and juiced

3 cups cabbage coleslaw mix with carrots

1. In a large skillet, heat the olive oil over medium heat.

2. Add the shallots and cook for 3 minutes, stirring, until softened.

3. Add the sole fillets and sprinkle with the chili powder. Cook for 3 to 5 minutes, stirring gently, until the fish flakes when tested with a fork. Remove the skillet from the heat.

4. Drizzle the lime zest and juice over the fish.

5. Serve with the coleslaw in tacos or over rice.

Increase Protein Tip: To make this a medium-protein recipe, add one more 6-ounce sole fillet. The protein content will increase to 18g per serving.

Ingredient Tip: If you like spicy food, you can add 1 diced medium jalapeño pepper to the shallots or add ½ teaspoon of red pepper flakes to the fish mixture along with the lime juice and zest.

Per Serving Calories: 176; Total fat: 9g; Saturated fat: 1g; Sodium: 315mg; Phosphorus: 265mg; Potassium: 451mg; Carbohydrates: 14g; Fiber: 4g; Protein: 13g; Sugar: 6g

Ginger Shrimp with Snow Peas

DIABETES-FRIENDLY, HIGH PROTEIN

Serves 4 / Prep Time: 20 minutes / Cook Time: 12 minutes

Ginger has a long culinary history because of its wonderful reputation for improving many health conditions due to its antibacterial properties. Ginger is a root vegetable that can be purchased as a root or as a ground powder in the spice aisle. It adds a wonderful warmth and spice to any recipe. This classic recipe is made with two types of peas.

2 tablespoons extra-virgin olive oil

1 tablespoon minced peeled
   fresh ginger

2 cups snow peas

1½ cups frozen baby peas

3 tablespoons water

1 pound medium shrimp, shelled
   and deveined

2 tablespoons low-sodium
   soy sauce

⅛ teaspoon freshly ground
   black pepper

1. In a large wok or skillet, heat the olive oil over medium heat.

2. Add the ginger and stir-fry for 1 to 2 minutes, until the ginger is fragrant.

3. Add the snow peas and stir-fry for 2 to 3 minutes, until they are tender-crisp.

4. Add the baby peas and the water and stir. Cover the wok and steam for 2 to 3 minutes or until the vegetables are tender.

5. Stir in the shrimp and stir-fry for 3 to 4 minutes, or until the shrimp have curled and turned pink.

6. Add the soy sauce and pepper; stir and serve.

Ingredient Tip: Snow peas can have a tough string along one side that won't soften very well during the stir-fry process. Just pinch the curly end of the pod and pull to remove it. Discard the string.

Per Serving Calories: 237; Total fat: 7g; Saturated fat: 1g; Sodium: 469mg; Phosphorus: 350mg; Potassium: 504mg; Carbohydrates: 12g; Fiber: 4g; Protein: 32g; Sugar: 5g

Roasted Cod with Plums

Serves 4 / Prep Time: 10 minutes / Cook Time: 20 minutes

Cod is a readily available mild and tender fish. But it can be a little boring by itself, so we need to add some oomph to take it up a notch. Plums are the perfect solution to bring the party to the plate. When roasted with the sole, plums add a rich flavor, texture, and color, changing a simple dish from bland to grand.

6 red plums, halved and pitted

1½ pounds cod fillets

3 tablespoons extra-virgin olive oil

2 tablespoons freshly squeezed
lemon juice

½ teaspoon dried thyme leaves

⅛ teaspoon salt

⅛ teaspoon freshly ground
black pepper

¾ cup plain whole-milk yogurt,
for serving

1. Preheat the oven to 375°F. Line a baking sheet with parchment paper.

2. Arrange the plums, cut-side up, along with the fish on the prepared baking sheet. Drizzle with the olive oil and lemon juice and sprinkle with the thyme, salt, and pepper.

3. Roast for 15 to 20 minutes or until the fish flakes when tested with a fork and the plums are tender.

4. Serve with the yogurt.

Ingredient Tip: There's no need to measure out exactly 2 tablespoons of lemon juice. A standard-size lemon has approximately 2 tablespoons juice in it. Simply squeeze all the juice from the lemon, being careful to avoid squeezing in the seeds.

Per Serving Calories: 230; Total fat: 9g; Saturated fat: 2g; Sodium: 154mg; Phosphorus: 197mg; Potassium: 437mg; Carbohydrates: 10g; Fiber: 1g; Protein: 27g; Sugar: 8g

Lemon Chicken

DIABETES-FRIENDLY, GLUTEN-FREE, MEDIUM PROTEIN

Serves 4 / Prep Time: 20 minutes / Cook Time: 24 minutes

Lemon chicken is the perfect balance of "simple enough to make on a weeknight" and "delicious enough to serve to company." The lemon juice's bright and tart flavor pairs beautifully with the olive oil, chicken, and vegetables in this quick and easy recipe.

2 lemons	⅛ teaspoon freshly ground
12 ounces boneless skinless chicken	black pepper
breasts, cubed	½ large onion, chopped
2 tablespoons extra-virgin olive oil	1 cup 2-inch green bean pieces
⅛ teaspoon salt	1 cup 2-inch asparagus pieces

1. Zest one of the lemons and place the zest into a medium bowl. Juice that lemon and add the juice to the bowl. Slice the remaining lemon, remove the seeds, and set aside.

2. In the bowl with the lemon juice, place the cubed chicken and set aside for 10 minutes to marinate.

3. When ready to cook, in a large skillet, heat the olive oil over medium heat.

4. Using a slotted spoon, remove the chicken from the lemon juice, reserving the lemon juice mixture. Add the chicken to the pan and cook for 3 to 4 minutes, stirring, until the chicken is lightly browned. It doesn't have to be completely cooked. Transfer the chicken to a clean plate and sprinkle with the salt and pepper.

5. Add the sliced lemon to the skillet and cook for 3 minutes on each side, turning once, until it is slightly caramelized. Transfer to the plate with the chicken.

6. Add the onion to the skillet and cook for 3 to 4 minutes, until the onion is tender-crisp, stirring to loosen the chicken drippings from the skillet.

7. Add the green beans and sauté for 2 minutes. Add the asparagus and sauté for 1 minute.

8. Return the chicken to the skillet and add the reserved lemon juice. Simmer for 4 to 6 minutes or until the chicken is thoroughly cooked to 165°F, the vegetables are tender, and the sauce has slightly thickened.

9. Add the caramelized lemon slices to the skillet and cook for 1 to 2 minutes, stirring, until hot. Serve.

Ingredient Tip: This recipe is delicious served over cooked brown rice or couscous. Serve about ½ cup of cooked grains per person.

Increase Protein Tip: To make this a high-protein recipe, omit the green beans and asparagus and replace with 1½ cups of frozen, shelled edamame.

Per Serving Calories: 207; Total fat: 9g; Saturated fat: 1g; Sodium: 121mg; Phosphorus: 245mg; Potassium: 593mg; Carbohydrates: 11g; Fiber: 4g; Protein: 22g; Sugar: 5g

Curried Chicken Stir-Fry

DIABETES-FRIENDLY, GLUTEN-FREE, MEDIUM PROTEIN

Serves 6 / Prep Time: 20 minutes / Cook Time: 15 minutes

It's great when most of the prep work for your recipe is already done, and you didn't have to do it. That's what happens when you open a jar of curry powder to make chicken curry. All the amazing spices such as cinnamon, chili powder, cumin, ginger, and turmeric have been blended together for you. All you have to do is toss it on the chicken.

12 ounces boneless skinless chicken breasts, cut into 1-inch cubes

2 teaspoons curry powder

⅛ teaspoon salt

⅛ teaspoon freshly ground black pepper

1 (20-ounce) can pineapple tidbits, strained, reserving juice

2 tablespoons extra-virgin olive oil

1 yellow onion, chopped

2 red bell peppers, chopped

1. In a medium bowl, toss the chicken, curry powder, salt, and pepper and set aside.

2. In a small saucepan, heat the reserved pineapple juice over low heat. Let it reduce, stirring occasionally, while you make the rest of the stir-fry.

3. In a large skillet, heat the olive oil over medium heat. Add the chicken. Stir-fry for 3 for 4 minutes or until the chicken is light brown; it doesn't have to completely cook. Transfer the chicken to a plate.

4. Add the onion to the skillet and cook for 3 minutes, stirring, until the onion is crisp-tender. Check to make sure the pineapple liquid isn't burning and continue to stir it. Add the bell peppers and stir-fry for another 3 minutes, until crisp tender.

5. Return the chicken to the skillet, add the pineapple tidbits and cook, stirring, for 3 to 4 minutes or until the chicken is cooked through.

6. Add the thickened pineapple juice to the skillet and stir. Serve.

Increase Protein Tip: To make this a high-protein recipe, increase the chicken to 1 pound. The protein content will increase to 25g per serving.

Per Serving Calories: 215; Total fat: 7g; Saturated fat: 1g; Sodium: 98mg; Phosphorus: 146mg; Potassium: 374mg; Carbohydrates: 19g; Fiber: 2g; Protein: 19g; Sugar: 16g

Thai-Style Chicken Salad

DIABETES-FRIENDLY, GLUTEN-FREE, HIGH PROTEIN

Serves 6 / Prep Time: 10 minutes

Thai recipes often include ingredients such as cilantro, lime, peanuts, hot chile peppers, and cabbage. Sometimes, the ingredient lists can be daunting and cumbersome to make. This recipe simplifies things with a total prep time of 10 minutes. You can omit the chile peppers for a milder flavor suitable for everyone. The zesty lime juice and crunchy salad bring a fresh and exciting flavor to the chicken. Try this salad in a wrap or serve it over a bed of lettuce.

3 cups shredded cooked chicken
  (about 1 pound)
1 (10-ounce) package shredded
  cabbage with carrots
2 limes

⅓ cup extra-virgin olive oil
¼ cup peanut butter
¼ teaspoon freshly ground
  black pepper
¼ cup chopped peanuts

1. In a large bowl, combine the chicken and cabbage and toss to mix.
2. In a small bowl, zest one of the limes. Juice both of the limes into the bowl. Add the olive oil, peanut butter, and pepper and mix with a whisk.
3. Drizzle the dressing over the salad and toss. Top with the peanuts and serve.

Ingredient Tip: If you like spicy food, add 1 or 2 minced jalapeño peppers to this salad. You could also add minced chipotle peppers in adobo sauce; just a teaspoon of each will add lots of heat.

Per Serving Calories: 415; Total fat: 31g; Saturated fat: 5g; Sodium: 119mg; Phosphorus: 239mg; Potassium: 408mg; Carbohydrates: 9g; Fiber: 3g; Protein: 28g; Sugar: 3g

Chicken Casserole

DIABETES-FRIENDLY, MEDIUM PROTEIN

Serves 6 / Prep Time: 30 minutes / Cook Time: 75 minutes

This chicken casserole dish is comforting and nutritious. Chicken stock is made first, followed by the chicken and vegetable mixture. The casserole is topped with crushed cereal for texture. Chicken thighs have more flavor to offer compared to chicken breasts; this is thanks to their slightly higher fat content. Chicken thighs are usually cheaper than breasts. More flavor for less money—it's a win-win!

2 tablespoons extra-virgin olive oil

6 bone-in skin-on chicken thighs

1 yellow onion, chopped

2½ cups plus ⅓ cup water

¼ teaspoon salt

3 cups frozen mixed vegetables

3 tablespoons flour

⅛ teaspoon freshly ground black pepper

1 cup crushed crisp rice cereal

1. In a large saucepan, heat the olive oil over medium heat.

2. Add the chicken thighs, skin-side down. Brown the skin thoroughly, moving the chicken around from time to time when it no longer sticks to the pan. This should take 12 to 15 minutes.

3. Remove the chicken from the skillet. Add the onion; cook and stir for 2 minutes to loosen the pan drippings.

4. Return the chicken to the skillet and add 2½ cups of water and the salt. Bring to a simmer, then reduce the heat to low and simmer for 30 to 40 minutes, stirring occasionally, until the chicken reaches 165°F and the juices run clear.

5. Remove the chicken from the saucepan and let cool for 10 minutes, while keeping the broth simmering. Then remove the meat from the skin and bones. Discard the skin and bones; shred the meat and return to the saucepan.

6. Add the frozen vegetables and bring to a simmer. Simmer for 3 to 5 minutes, stirring occasionally, or until the vegetables are thawed.

7. Combine the flour with the remaining ⅓ cup of water and pepper; mix well. Stir into the saucepan and simmer for 3 to 5 minutes or until the sauce has thickened.

CONTINUES NEXT PAGE

8. Preheat the oven to 400°F.

9. Pour the chicken mixture into a 2-quart baking dish and top with the cereal.

10. Bake for 20 to 25 minutes, or until the filling is bubbling and the cereal is lightly browned. Serve.

Increase Protein Tip: To make this a high-protein recipe, use 8 bone-in, skin-on chicken thighs. The protein content will increase to 28 grams per serving.

Per Serving Calories: 203; Total fat: 9g; Saturated fat: 2g; Sodium: 181mg; Phosphorus: 178mg; Potassium: 264mg; Carbohydrates: 9g; Fiber: 2g; Protein: 21g; Sugar: 1g

Chicken Patties with Dill

DIABETES-FRIENDLY, GLUTEN-FREE, HIGH PROTEIN

Serves 4 / Prep Time: 25 minutes / Cook Time: 20 minutes

Chicken patties are an old-fashioned recipe with a flavor that never goes out of style. Grated vegetables are added to ground chicken, then sautéed in heart-healthy olive oil for a crisp patty that is tender and moist on the inside. As animal protein goes, chicken is a good option for dialysis patients because it is lower in potassium and phosphorus compared to other sources.

3 tablespoons extra-virgin olive oil, divided

1 large carrot, finely grated or diced

1 yellow onion, grated or diced

½ cup puffed rice cereal, crushed

1 teaspoon dried dill weed

Pinch salt

⅛ teaspoon freshly ground black pepper

1 pound lean ground chicken

1. In a large skillet, heat 1 tablespoon of olive oil over medium heat.

2. Add the carrot and onion and cook for 4 to 6 minutes, until tender. Add the crushed cereal, dill, salt, and pepper and stir. Transfer the vegetable mixture into a medium bowl and let cool for 15 minutes. Do not wipe out or wash the skillet.

3. Add the ground chicken to the vegetables and work gently but thoroughly with your hands until combined.

4. Form the chicken mixture into 4 patties and place onto a plate and freeze for 10 minutes, so they firm up and are easier to work with.

5. In the same skillet, heat the remaining 2 tablespoons of olive oil over medium heat. Add the chicken patties; cook for 6 to 7 minutes per side, turning once, until the patties reach 165°F and the juices run clear. Serve.

Per Serving Calories: 311; Total fat: 15g; Saturated fat: 3g; Sodium: 140 mg; Phosphorus: 262mg; Potassium: 389mg; Carbohydrates: 6g; Fiber: 1g; Protein: 36g; Sugar: 2g

Chicken and Cabbage Stir-Fry

Serves 4 / Prep Time: 20 minutes / Cook Time: 20 minutes

This recipe tastes like the inside of an egg roll! Stir-fry recipes like this one are ideal for busy weeknights. There's not much preparation involved because you use a cabbage coleslaw blend. Cabbage is a popular ingredient in this book—and for good reason. A cruciferous vegetable, cabbage is highly nutritious yet happens to be low in potassium. Cabbage is also a very economical vegetable, so it's good for both your health and your wallet!

2 tablespoons extra-virgin olive oil

8 ounces boneless skinless chicken breasts, cubed

1 yellow onion, chopped

1 red bell pepper, chopped

1 (16-ounce) package cabbage coleslaw blend with carrots

⅓ cup water

2 tablespoons low-sodium soy sauce

1. In a large skillet, heat the olive oil over medium heat.
2. Add the chicken and stir-fry for 5 to 6 minutes, or until the chicken is cooked through. Transfer the chicken to a plate and set aside.
3. Add the onion to the skillet and stir-fry for 3 to 4 minutes, or until crisp-tender, scraping the pan to loosen any bits.
4. Add the bell pepper and stir-fry for another 2 minutes, until crisp-tender.
5. Add the coleslaw mix and stir-fry for 3 to 5 minutes longer, until softened.
6. Return the chicken to the skillet along with the water and soy sauce and stir-fry for 3 to 5 minutes longer, or until the sauce is slightly thickened and the vegetables are tender. Serve.

Increase Protein Tip: To make this a high-protein recipe, only use half of the coleslaw blend and increase the chicken to ¾ pound. The protein content will increase to 28g per serving.

Per Serving Calories: 206; Total fat: 9g; Saturated fat: 2g; Sodium: 413mg; Phosphorus: 173mg; Potassium: 621mg; Carbohydrates: 13g; Fiber: 4g; Protein: 20g; Sugar: 6g

Slow Cooker Chicken with Apple and Onions

GLUTEN-FREE, HIGH PROTEIN

Serves 4 / Prep Time: 15 minutes / Cook Time: 6 hours

Have you ever ended up with an abundance of apples for any reason? In addition to sweet dishes like apple pie, apple crisp, and applesauce, there are also savory recipes that use apples, such as this delicious slow-cooker chicken recipe. The tart and sweet flavor of Granny Smith apples tastes amazing when combined with mustard, honey, and onions.

---

1 large yellow onion, chopped

6 boneless skinless chicken thighs,
   cut into strips

3 Granny Smith apples, sliced

2 tablespoons Dijon mustard

2 tablespoons honey

⅛ teaspoon salt

⅛ teaspoon freshly ground
   black pepper

---

1. In a 4- or 5-quart slow cooker, place the onions. Top with the chicken, then the apples.

2. In a small bowl, combine the mustard, honey, salt, and pepper and mix well. Pour the mixture over the ingredients in the slow cooker.

3. Cover and cook on low for 6 hours or on high for 3 hours, or until the chicken is cooked through and the apples and onions are tender. Serve.

Appliance Tip: To cook this recipe on the stovetop, add 2 tablespoons of olive oil. Heat the olive oil in a saucepan and add the onion; cook and stir for 3 minutes. Add the chicken; cook and stir until lightly browned, about 5 minutes. Then add the apple and the mustard-honey mixture. Simmer over low heat for 15 to 20 minutes, or until the chicken is cooked through.

Per Serving Calories: 309; Total fat: 7g; Saturated fat: 2g; Sodium: 369mg; Phosphorus: 258mg; Potassium: 465mg; Carbohydrates: 30g; Fiber: 4g; Protein: 30g; Sugar: 22g

Chicken with Apricots

DIABETES-FRIENDLY, GLUTEN-FREE, HIGH PROTEIN

Serves 4 / Prep Time: 15 minutes / Cook Time: 15 minutes

Apricots are sweet and sour, and the perfect complement to tender and savory chicken. Fresh apricots are in season in the summer and can be hard to find year-round. This recipe uses canned apricots, and the juice makes the sauce. Serve this dish with some cooked couscous or rice.

---

1 (15-ounce) can canned apricot halves, strained, reserving juice, divided

12 ounces boneless skinless chicken breasts, cubed

⅛ teaspoon salt

⅛ teaspoon freshly ground black pepper

2 tablespoons extra-virgin olive oil

1 yellow onion, chopped

1 cup green beans

---

1. In a food processor or blender, combine four apricot halves with the juice from the can; process until smooth and set aside.

2. Sprinkle the chicken with salt and pepper.

3. In a large skillet, heat the olive oil over medium heat and add the chicken; cook until lightly browned, stirring occasionally for 3 to 5 minutes. Remove the chicken from the skillet and set aside.

4. Add the onion to the skillet; cook and stir for 3 to 4 minutes or until crisp-tender. Add the green beans to the skillet; cook and stir for another 3 minutes, until crisp-tender.

5. Return the chicken to the skillet and add the apricot sauce mixture. Bring to a simmer and simmer for 4 to 6 minutes or until the chicken is cooked through.

6. Add the remaining apricots to the skillet and heat through. Serve.

Reduce Protein Tip: To make this recipe medium-protein, reduce the chicken breasts to 8 ounces. The protein will decrease to 19g per serving. Feel free to add another bell pepper to increase bulk.

Per Serving Calories: 256; Total fat: 10g; Saturated fat: 2g; Sodium: 127mg; Phosphorus: 256mg; Potassium: 598mg; Carbohydrates: 17g; Fiber: 3g; Protein: 27g; Sugar: 13g

Herbed Chicken and Veggies

DIABETES-FRIENDLY, GLUTEN-FREE, HIGH PROTEIN

Serves 6 / Prep Time: 25 minutes / Cook Time: 7 hours

When cooked in a slow cooker, chicken breasts can end up dry and overcooked. Chicken thighs, however, cook beautifully in this appliance. Sweet potatoes and carrots not only provide wonderful color to this recipe, they are also both excellent sources of beta-carotene, an antioxidant and precursor to vitamin A found only in plants. This hearty and savory dish is perfect for a cold winter night. Hard root vegetables are put into the bottom of a slow cooker because they take longer to cook. The meat is put on top so it cooks more slowly and gently.

4 large carrots, peeled and sliced

2 sweet potatoes, peeled and cubed

1 yellow onion, chopped

6 boneless skinless chicken thighs, cut into strips (about 24 ounces)

1 teaspoon dried Italian seasoning

⅛ teaspoon salt

⅛ teaspoon freshly ground black pepper

⅓ cup water

1. In a 4 to 5 quart slow cooker, combine the carrots, potatoes, and onion.

2. Sprinkle the chicken with Italian seasoning, salt, and pepper and place on top of the vegetables in the slow cooker. Add the water.

3. Cover and cook on low for 5 to 7 hours. Stir and serve.

Reduce Protein Tip: To make this a medium-protein recipe, use 16 ounces of chicken thighs. The protein content will decrease to 22g per serving.

Per Serving Calories: 261; Total fat: 7g; Saturated fat: 2g; Sodium: 227mg; Phosphorus: 283mg; Potassium: 587mg; Carbohydrates: 15g; Fiber: 3g; Protein: 33g; Sugar: 5g

Pork Tenderloin with Roasted Fruit

GLUTEN-FREE, MEDIUM PROTEIN

Serves 4 / Prep Time: 20 minutes / Cook Time: 25 minutes

Fruit pairs very well with meat, especially moist and mild meat such as pork tenderloin. The meat and fruit roast in the oven, concentrating the fruit's sweetness and caramelizing the pork. Despite what is commonly thought, pork is not the "other white meat." Like beef, pork is a red meat, and thus it should be considered an indulgent food eaten only on occasion.

2 tablespoons extra-virgin olive oil

1 chopped red onion

2 pears, seeded and cut into ½-inch wedges

1 (12-ounce) pork tenderloin, cut into 1-inch strips

⅛ teaspoon salt

⅛ teaspoon freshly ground black pepper

1½ cups red grapes

1 teaspoon dried thyme leaves

1. Preheat the oven to 400°F.

2. Drizzle the olive oil onto a rimmed baking sheet. Add the onion and pears; toss to coat. Roast for 10 minutes.

3. Remove the pan from the oven and add the pork. Sprinkle with the salt and pepper. Add the grapes and sprinkle everything with the thyme; stir gently.

4. Arrange the fruit and pork in a single layer.

5. Roast, uncovered, stirring gently once during cooking time, for 13 to 18 minutes or until the fruit is tender and the pork registers at least 150°F with a food thermometer. Stir and serve.

Diabetes Tip: To reduce the chance of a blood sugar spike, omit the fruit and roast the pork with your favorite vegetables instead.

Per Serving Calories: 283; Total fat: 10g; Saturated fat: 2g; Sodium: 128mg; Phosphorus: 258mg; Potassium: 612mg; Carbohydrates: 27g; Fiber: 4g; Protein: 23g; Sugar: 19g

Rice-Stuffed Mini Meatloaves

DIABETES-FRIENDLY, GLUTEN-FREE, HIGH PROTEIN

Makes 5 mini loaves / Prep Time: 20 minutes / Cook Time: 50 minutes

This easy stuffed meatloaf recipe is a nice change of pace from the traditional larger meatloaf. You can make these little meatloaves ahead of time and store them in the fridge; bake them just before serving. Each of these meatloaves contain a whopping 4 milligrams of iron.

Olive oil cooking spray	1 large egg yolk
1½ cups water, plus 2 tablespoons	3 tablespoons mustard, divided
10 tablespoons uncooked brown rice	Pinch salt
	Pinch freshly ground black pepper
1¼ pounds extra-lean ground beef	½ cup sour cream

1. Preheat the oven to 350°F. Spray a 6-cup muffin tin with cooking spray and set aside.

2. In a medium saucepan, combine the water and brown rice over medium heat. Bring to a boil, then reduce the heat, cover, and simmer for 25 to 30 minutes or until the rice is tender. Drain if necessary and set aside to cool for 20 minutes.

3. Meanwhile, in a medium bowl, combine the ground beef, egg yolk, 1 tablespoon of mustard, the salt, and pepper and mix well. Divide the beef mixture into 5 balls and press into the prepared cups against the sides and bottom, making a "crust," leaving a space for the filling.

4. In a small bowl, combine the remaining 2 tablespoons of mustard with the sour cream and mix them together. Add the sour cream mixture to the rice and mix them together. Spoon about ¼ cup of the rice mixture into the center of the beef cups. Put 2 tablespoons of water in the empty muffin cup.

5. Bake the meatloaves for 22 to 27 minutes or until a food thermometer inserted into the center reads 160°F and the juices run clear. Let cool for 5 minutes, then carefully remove from the muffin tins and serve.

Per Serving (1 meatloaf) Calories: 344; Total fat: 14g; Saturated fat: 6g; Sodium: 210mg; Phosphorus: 338mg; Potassium: 462mg; Carbohydrates: 19g; Fiber: 1g; Protein: 34g; Sugar: 1g

Vegetable Beef Stir-Fry

DIABETES-FRIENDLY, HIGH PROTEIN

Serves 4 / Prep Time: 10 minutes / Cook Time: 15 minutes

In a typical beef stir-fry recipe, the ratio of beef to vegetables is not ideal for a person with CKD. Most dishes, especially those prepared in a restaurant, contain at least 6 ounces of beef per serving and excessive amounts of sodium. This recipe changes that by limiting the beef to 3 ounces per serving and creating a sauce that is lower in sodium by using a reduced-sodium broth and soy sauce. This recipe is high in both protein and iron, making it ideal for dialysis patients.

¾ cup low-sodium vegetable broth

2 tablespoons cornstarch

2 tablespoons low-sodium soy sauce

12 ounces beef sirloin tip, cut into ½-inch strips

⅛ teaspoon salt

⅛ teaspoon freshly ground black pepper

2 tablespoons extra-virgin olive oil

1 (14-ounce) package frozen stir-fry vegetables

2 tablespoons water

1. In a small bowl, combine the broth, cornstarch, and soy sauce and whisk to combine. Sprinkle the beef with the salt and pepper.

2. In a wok or large skillet, heat the olive oil over medium heat. Add the beef and stir-fry for 3 to 4 minutes, or until browned. Remove the beef from the wok and set aside.

3. In the wok, add the stir-fry vegetables with the water and stir-fry until hot and cooked through.

4. Return the beef to the wok.

5. Stir the sauce again and add to the wok. Stir-fry until the sauce for 2 to 3 minutes, until it is bubbly and thickened. Serve.

Ingredient Tip: You don't have to use frozen vegetables in this recipe. Feel free to replace with your favorite combination of fresh vegetables. Water chestnuts, broccoli, carrots, and peppers are all good choices.

Per Serving Calories: 256; Total fat: 11g; Saturated fat: 2g; Sodium: 466mg; Phosphorus: 288mg; Potassium: 534mg; Carbohydrates: 13g; Fiber: 3g; Protein: 28g; Sugar: 3g

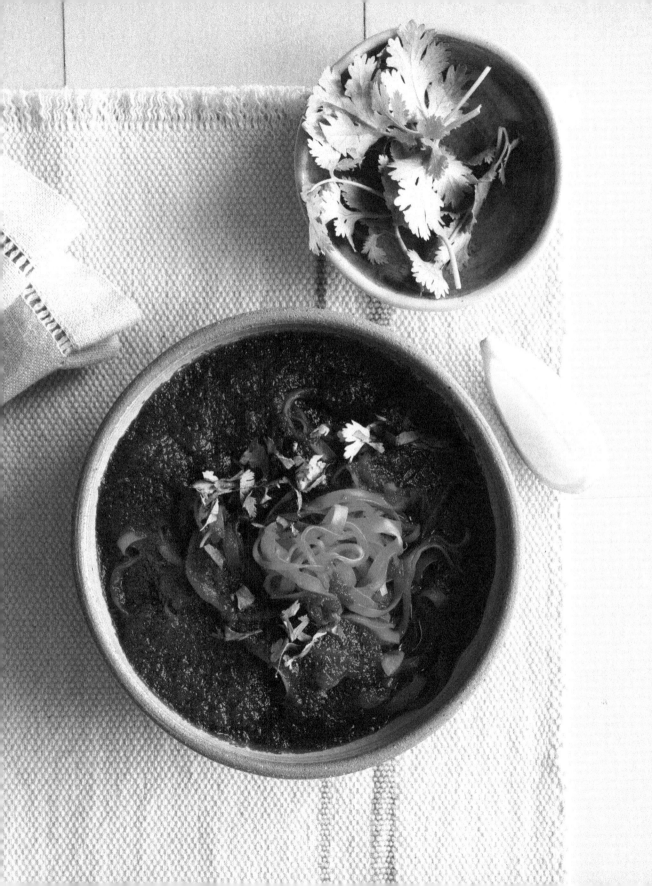

CHAPTER 6

Soups and Stews

⇦ *Thai-Style Beet Soup, page 110*

Vegetable Bisque

Serves 4 / Prep Time: 15 minutes / Cook Time: 30 minutes

A bisque is a soup that is pureed, then combined with cream to make a rich and smooth mixture that is hearty and soothing. Carrots, bell peppers, and mushrooms combine beautifully in this rich and comforting recipe. Cream cheese is added to this recipe to make it even more luxurious.

4 cups low-sodium vegetable broth
3 large carrots, sliced
1 yellow bell pepper, sliced
1 cup sliced button mushrooms
⅛ teaspoon salt

⅛ teaspoon freshly ground black pepper
1 (8-ounce) package cream cheese, cubed

1. In a heavy saucepan, combine the broth, carrots, bell pepper, mushrooms, salt, and pepper over medium heat. Bring to a boil, then reduce the heat to low.

2. Simmer for 20 to 25 minutes, or until the vegetables are very tender.

3. Using a slotted spoon, remove the vegetables from the broth and transfer them to a food processor. Add the cream cheese and process until smooth.

4. Return the pureed mixture to the broth in the saucepan and stir. Reheat for 3 to 5 minutes, until steaming. Do not boil. Serve.

Appliance Tip: You can cook this soup in the slow cooker. Combine the mushrooms, carrots, broth, salt, and pepper in a 3-quart slow cooker. Cover and cook on low for 6 to 8 hours or until the vegetables are tender. Puree the vegetables in a food processor with the cream cheese and cream as directed above, then return to the slow cooker. Heat on high for 30 minutes, then serve.

Per Serving Calories: 247; Total fat: 20g; Saturated fat: 12g; Sodium: 429mg; Phosphorus: 109mg; Potassium: 386mg; Carbohydrates: 14g; Fiber: 2g; Protein: 5g; Sugar: 7g

French Onion Soup

DIABETES-FRIENDLY, GLUTEN-FREE, HIGH FIBER, LOW PROTEIN, VEGETARIAN

Serves 4 / Prep Time: 25 minutes / Cook Time: 70 minutes

French onion soup is typically made with beef stock, but this can raise the recipe's phosphorus content. Using a good-quality or homemade vegetable stock will infuse your soup with healthy and delicious flavors, while still tasting robust. Instead of using bread and cheese to top the soup, sour cream is blended in for a rich and creamy texture.

2 tablespoons butter

1 tablespoon extra-virgin olive oil

3 large yellow onions, chopped

5 cups low-sodium vegetable broth

⅛ teaspoon salt

⅛ teaspoon freshly ground
   black pepper

1 cup sour cream

2 tablespoons cornstarch

1. In a large saucepan, melt the butter with the olive oil over medium heat. Add the onions, reduce the heat to medium low, and cook for about 30 minutes, stirring occasionally, until the onions are golden brown.

2. Add the broth, salt, and pepper and bring to a simmer. Simmer for 20 to 30 minutes.

3. In a medium bowl, whisk the sour cream and cornstarch.

4. Add 1 cup of the hot broth from the soup to the sour cream mixture and whisk together until smooth. This is called tempering and makes the sour cream blend into the soup without curdling.

5. Add the sour cream mixture back to the soup and stir. Reheat until steaming; do not boil. Serve.

Appliance Tip: You can make this recipe in a slow cooker. Brown the onions as directed, then transfer to a 3- to 4-quart slow cooker and add the broth, salt, and pepper. Cover and cook on low for 6 to 7 hours or on high for 3½ hours. Add the sour cream mixture as directed, then cook on high for 20 to 30 minutes or until hot.

Per Serving Calories: 269; Total fat: 21g; Saturated fat: 10g; Sodium: 314mg; Phosphorus: 87mg; Potassium: 292mg; Carbohydrates: 20g; Fiber: 2g; Protein: 3g; Sugar: 8g

Tomato-Free Slow Cooker White Chili

DIABETES-FRIENDLY, GLUTEN-FREE, HIGH FIBER, MEDIUM PROTEIN, VEGAN

Serves 6 / Prep Time: 20 minutes / Cook Time: 8 hours

There are many chili recipes, and while most are delicious, it can be hard to find a tomato-free recipe. Tomatoes are high in potassium, and when pureed to form a sauce or juice, the potassium may be more likely to raise your blood potassium level. This white chili is easy to make and hearty even without tomatoes. The kidney beans are double-boiled to reduce their potassium content by about half.

---

1 cup dried kidney beans, sorted and rinsed

6 cups low-sodium vegetable broth

1 yellow onion, chopped

4 garlic cloves, minced

2 tablespoons chili powder

⅛ teaspoon salt

⅛ teaspoon freshly ground black pepper

2 tablespoons extra-virgin olive oil

---

1. In a large saucepan, cover the beans with water and bring to a boil. Boil for 10 minutes. Drain the beans, discarding the water.

2. In a 4-quart slow cooker, combine the beans, broth, onion, garlic, chili powder, salt, and pepper.

3. Cover and cook on low for 6 to 8 hours or on high for 3 to 4 hours, or until the beans and rice are tender.

4. Transfer ½ cup of the beans from the slow cooker to a food processor or blender. Add the olive oil and puree. Return to the slow cooker. Heat on high for 20 minutes, then serve.

Appliance Tip: You can make this recipe on the stovetop. Boil the beans as directed, drain, then cover with fresh water again and bring to a simmer. Remove the pan from the heat and let the beans soak for 1 hour. Drain the beans again, then add all the remaining ingredients. Partially cover and simmer for 1½ hours or until the beans are tender.

Per Serving Calories: 171; Total fat: 5g; Saturated fat: 1g; Sodium: 271mg; Phosphorus: 148mg; Potassium: 561mg; Carbohydrates: 24g; Fiber: 9g; Protein: 8g; Sugar: 3g

Minestrone

DIABETES-FRIENDLY, HIGH FIBER, MEDIUM PROTEIN, VEGAN

Serves 4 / Prep Time: 20 minutes / Cook Time: 35 minutes

Originating in Italy, minestrone is really just a thick vegetable soup. This version includes orzo, a rice-shaped pasta. Whole-wheat orzo contains more fiber than regular orzo. If unavailable, you can use regular orzo or another whole-grain pasta of your choosing. For a French-inspired touch, add ½ teaspoon of dried Herbs de Provence or dried thyme along with the chicken broth.

2 tablespoons extra-virgin olive oil

1 yellow onion, chopped

2 large carrots, peeled and chopped

4 cups low-sodium vegetable broth

2 cups green beans, cut into
  2-inch pieces

⅛ teaspoon salt

⅛ teaspoon freshly ground
  black pepper

½ cup whole-wheat orzo pasta

1. In a large saucepan, heat the olive oil over medium heat.
2. Add the onion and cook for 3 to 4 minutes, stirring, until the onion starts to soften.
3. Add the carrots, cook, and stir for another 3 minutes.
4. Add the broth, green beans, salt, and pepper and bring to a simmer.
5. Reduce the heat to low and simmer for 15 to 20 minutes or until the vegetables are almost tender.
6. Add the pasta and bring back to a simmer. Simmer for 8 to 10 minutes or until the pasta is tender. Serve.

Increase Protein Tip: To make this a high-protein recipe, use low-sodium chicken broth instead of vegetable broth. The protein content will increase to 10 grams per serving.

Ingredient Tip: You can serve this recipe topped with Easy Pesto (page 151) or top with some grated Parmesan cheese for the perfect finishing touch.

Per Serving Calories: 190; Total fat: 8g; Saturated fat: 1g; Sodium: 243mg; Phosphorus: 113g; Potassium: 354mg; Carbohydrates: 27g; Fiber: 5g; Protein: 5g; Sugar: 5g

Roasted Carrot and Ginger Soup

DIABETES-FRIENDLY, GLUTEN-FREE, HIGH FIBER, LOW PROTEIN, VEGETARIAN

Serves 4 / Prep Time: 20 minutes / Cook Time: 50 minutes

Ginger brings warmth and spice to this simple soup made with roasted carrots and onions. Don't skip the roasting step—it brings about an incredible depth of flavor you won't be able to resist. Sour cream adds rich decadence to this dish, making it a perfect treat for lunch or a first course if you're serving guests.

6 large carrots, peeled and sliced

1 red onion, chopped

2 tablespoons extra-virgin olive oil

1 tablespoon minced peeled
   fresh ginger

⅛ teaspoon salt

⅛ teaspoon freshly ground
   black pepper

3½ cups water

½ cup pineapple-orange juice

½ cup sour cream

1. Preheat the oven to 400°F.

2. On a large rimmed baking sheet, place the carrots and onion and drizzle with the olive oil. Sprinkle with the ginger, salt, and pepper. Toss to coat.

3. Roast the vegetables for 30 to 35 minutes, stirring twice while they cook, until they are tender and lightly browned around the edges.

4. Transfer the vegetables to a large saucepan. Add the water and bring to a simmer. Simmer for 10 minutes or until the vegetables are soft.

5. In a food processor, puree the mixture in three separate batches because hot soup expands when blended. Return to the saucepan.

6. In a medium bowl, combine the pineapple-orange juice and sour cream and whisk together. Add 1 cup of the hot soup and whisk again. Stir into the soup and heat through; serve.

Ingredient Tip: To make this recipe vegan, omit the sour cream and add richness by topping the soup with a tablespoon of coconut cream. Coconut cream is available canned in most grocery stores.

Per Serving Calories: 173; Total fat: 13g; Saturated fat: 4g; Sodium: 315mg; Phosphorus: 68mg; Potassium: 429mg; Carbohydrates: 15g; Fiber: 4g; Protein: 2g; Sugar: 7g

Roasted Onion Clam Chowder

GLUTEN-FREE, HIGH FIBER, HIGH PROTEIN

Serves 6 / Prep Time: 20 minutes / Cook Time: 1 hour

A chowder is a thick soup that is usually made with potatoes for texture. In this version of clam chowder, onions and garlic are roasted to make them very sweet and tender. The potatoes are double-boiled to reduce potassium, and a few of the potatoes are mashed when cooked to thicken the chowder.

---

2 russet potatoes, peeled and cubed

2 yellow onions, chopped

8 whole unpeeled garlic cloves

2 tablespoons extra-virgin olive oil

4 cups low-sodium chicken stock

⅛ teaspoon salt

⅛ teaspoon freshly ground black pepper

1 (10-ounce) can clams

---

1. Place the potatoes in a large saucepan, cover with water, and bring to a boil on high heat. Boil for 10 minutes, then drain the potatoes and discard the water.

2. Preheat the oven to 400°F.

3. On a rimmed baking sheet, combine the onions, garlic, and olive oil. Roast for 30 to 35 minutes, stirring once during the cooking time, until they are tender and light golden brown around the edges. Squeeze the garlic to remove the skins. Discard the skins and set the garlic and onions aside.

4. In the same saucepan, combine the potatoes, chicken stock, salt, and pepper and bring to a boil over medium heat. Reduce the heat to low and simmer for 20 to 25 minutes or until the potatoes are tender.

5. Using a potato masher, mash half of the potatoes, leaving some whole for a chunky texture.

6. Add the onions and garlic to the saucepan along with the clams and their juices. Simmer for 5 to 10 minutes or until hot. Serve.

Diabetes Tip: To make this a diabetes-friendly recipe, omit the potatoes, skip step 1, and use 2 parsnips instead. The carbohydrate content will decrease to 18g per serving.

Per Serving Calories: 216; Total fat: 6g; Saturated fat: 1g; Sodium: 141mg; Phosphorus: 205mg; Potassium: 565mg; Carbohydrates: 29g; Fiber: 3g; Protein: 13g; Sugar: 3g

Chicken Parmesan Soup

DIABETES-FRIENDLY, HIGH FIBER, HIGH PROTEIN

Serves 4 / Prep Time: 20 minutes / Cook Time: 7 hours

Traditional chicken Parmesan is a comfort food that is far from ideal for the renal diet because it has a lot of sodium, phosphorus, and potassium. This recipe offers the flavors of chicken Parmesan while keeping the relevant nutrients at acceptable levels. The slow cooker makes preparation a breeze and creates delicious, tender chicken. Regular boneless skinless chicken breast can somewhat dry out when prepared in a slow cooker, so be sure to use bone in.

1 leek, chopped

2 tablespoons extra-virgin olive oil

2 (6-ounce) bone-in, skin-on chicken breasts

2 cups frozen corn

4 cups water, divided

2 tablespoons tomato paste

⅛ teaspoon salt

⅛ teaspoon freshly ground black pepper

3 tablespoons grated Parmesan cheese

1. Place the leek in a 3- to 4-quart slow cooker.

2. In a large saucepan, heat the olive oil over medium heat. Add the chicken breasts, skin-side down, and cook for 8 to 10 minutes, until well-browned.

3. Place the chicken in the slow cooker and top with the corn.

4. In the same saucepan used to brown the chicken, combine 1 cup of water and the tomato paste and bring to a simmer, scraping up the brown bits. Pour into the slow cooker along with the remaining 3 cups of water, the salt, and pepper.

5. Cover and cook on low for 6 to 7 hours.

6. Remove the chicken from the soup and let cool for 15 minutes. Remove the skin and bones and discard. Shred the chicken, then return it to the soup.

7. Cook on high for 10 minutes, then serve topped with cheese.

Ingredient Tip: Feel free to add more fresh or dried herbs or spices to this recipe. Basil, oregano, and parsley are all excellent possibilities.

Per Serving Calories: 323; Total fat: 15g; Saturated fat: 4g; Sodium: 226mg; Phosphorus: 233mg; Potassium: 441mg; Carbohydrates: 21g; Fiber: 3g; Protein: 28g; Sugar: 5g

Slow Cooker Potato Leek Soup

GLUTEN-FREE, HIGH FIBER, HIGH PROTEIN

Serves 4 / Prep Time: 15 minutes / Cook Time: 8 hours

This classic soup is made in a slow cooker. The potatoes are double-boiled before they are cooked, thus reducing their potassium content by about 50 percent. Leeks are a good source of quercetin, an antioxidant with anti-inflammatory potential in the body. Make sure to add the chives at the end or else the heat of cooking will reduce their delicate onion flavor.

2 large russet potatoes, peeled and chopped

5 cups low-sodium chicken broth

2 leeks, rinsed and chopped

⅛ teaspoon salt

⅛ teaspoon freshly ground black pepper

1 cup heavy cream

2 tablespoons minced chives

1. Place the potatoes in a large saucepan, cover with water, and bring to a boil on high heat. Boil for 10 minutes, then drain the potatoes and discard the water.

2. In the slow cooker, combine the potatoes, broth, leeks, salt, and pepper. Cover and cook on low for 6 to 8 hours.

3. Add the cream to the slow cooker. Using an immersion blender or potato masher, blend or mash the vegetables to make a smooth soup. You can also puree the vegetables in a food processor; do them half at a time, then return to the slow cooker.

4. Heat the soup for 20 minutes on high, then serve, garnished with the chives.

Ingredient Tip: Leeks can be very sandy, so after you cut off the root end and about 3 inches of the green part, cut the leeks in half. Rinse them under cool, running water, making sure to separate the leaves to get out all the sand. Then chop and continue with the recipe.

Reduce Protein Tip: To make this a medium-protein recipe, replace the chicken broth with low-sodium vegetable broth. The protein content will decrease to 7g per serving.

Per Serving Calories: 395; Total fat: 24g; Saturated fat: 14g; Sodium: 201mg; Phosphorus: 243mg; Potassium: 599mg; Carbohydrates: 45g; Fiber: 3g; Protein: 12g; Sugar: 5g

Thai-Style Beet Soup

GLUTEN-FREE, HIGH FIBER, MEDIUM PROTEIN

Serves 4 / Prep Time: 15 minutes / Cook Time: 35 minutes

If you want a break from the traditional, this Thai-style beet soup is for you. In addition to contributing beautiful color, beets are also wonderfully nutritious. One beet provides nearly a quarter of your daily folate needs, an essential vitamin many people are deficient in. You can also use golden beets in this recipe. If you're not a cilantro fan, feel free to replace it with basil.

---

2 tablespoons extra-virgin olive oil

3 medium beets, scrubbed, peeled, and chopped

5 cups water

2 tablespoons yellow curry paste

⅛ teaspoon salt

⅛ teaspoon freshly ground black pepper

8 ounces thin rice noodles

1 lime, zested and juiced

3 tablespoons chopped fresh cilantro

---

1. In a large saucepan, heat the olive oil over medium heat.

2. Add the beets and cook for 3 to 4 minutes while stirring. Add the water and yellow curry paste. Bring to a boil over medium heat. Then cover the pan, reduce the heat to low, and simmer for about 25 minutes, until the beets are tender.

3. In a food processor, puree the soup in two or three batches or use an immersion blender or potato masher directly in the saucepan. Bring the soup back to a simmer over low heat, stirring occasionally.

4. To prepare the rice noodles, bring a large pot of water to a boil over high heat. Using tongs, add the noodles and submerge. When the noodles are tender, 1 to 2 minutes, drain. If you are using flat noodles, it may take 8 to 10 minutes for the noodles to soften.

5. Divide the soup among bowls and top with the noodles. Drizzle with the lime juice and zest, and sprinkle with the cilantro before serving.

Per Serving Calories: 302; Total fat: 7g; Saturated fat: 1g; Sodium: 364mg; Phosphorus: 119mg; Potassium: 268mg; Carbohydrates: 54g; Fiber: 3g; Protein: 5g; Sugar: 5g

Turkey and Corn Chowder

DIABETES-FRIENDLY, GLUTEN-FREE, HIGH FIBER, HIGH PROTEIN

Serves 6 / Prep Time: 20 minutes / Cook Time: 35 minutes

This rich and hearty soup contains potatoes, but they are double-boiled to reduce potassium. Heavy cream contains almost 50 percent less phosphorus compared to skim milk, and it adds an irresistible richness to this soup.

2 russet potatoes, peeled
  and chopped
2 tablespoons extra-virgin olive oil
1 onion, chopped
4 cups water
1½ cups frozen yellow corn

⅛ teaspoon salt
⅛ teaspoon freshly ground
  black pepper
2 cups shredded cooked turkey
  or chicken
1 cup heavy cream

1. Place the potatoes in a large saucepan, cover with water, and bring to a boil on high heat. Boil for 10 minutes, then drain the potatoes and discard the water.

2. In a large saucepan, heat the olive oil over medium heat. Add the onion and cook for 3 to 4 minutes, stirring until tender.

3. Add the water, corn, potatoes, salt, and pepper and bring to a simmer.

4. Reduce the heat to low and simmer for 20 to 25 minutes or until the potatoes are tender. Remove half the vegetables from the soup and puree. Return to the soup.

5. Add the turkey and cream to the soup. Heat over medium heat until steaming; do not boil. Serve.

Appliance Tip: You can make this recipe in the slow cooker. Boil the potatoes as directed, then omit the oil. Combine the onion, corn, water, potatoes, salt, and pepper in a 3- or 4- quart slow cooker. Cover and cook on low for 6 hours or on high for 3 hours. Then mash about half the veggies in the crockpot, add the cream and turkey, and heat on high for 10 minutes.

Per Serving Calories: 307; Total fat: 20g; Saturated fat: 10g; Sodium: 110mg; Phosphorus: 181mg; Potassium: 407mg; Carbohydrates: 16g; Fiber: 2g; Protein: 17g; Sugar: 3g

Hearty Veggie Stew

DIABETES-FRIENDLY, GLUTEN-FREE, HIGH FIBER, LOW PROTEIN, VEGAN

Serves 4 / Prep Time: 20 minutes / Cook Time: 6 to 8 hours

A slow cooker is the ideal cooking vessel for a stew. The appliance really brings out the vegetables' flavor. Some people are concerned that the long cooking time required in slow cooker recipes could decrease the veggies' nutritional value. The truth is quite the opposite. Slow cooking uses a lower cooking temperature than regular cooking, so the nutrients are actually better preserved compared to high-heat cooking. Baby peas are also called petite peas; either will work for this recipe. Feel free to experiment with other vegetables when making this stew.

1 large sweet potato, peeled
   and chopped
5 cups water
2 cups baby carrots
2 cups chopped celery
1 yellow onion, chopped

⅛ teaspoon salt
⅛ teaspoon freshly ground
   black pepper
2 cups frozen baby peas
4 tablespoons extra-virgin olive oil

1. Place the sweet potato in a large saucepan, cover with water, and bring to a boil on high heat. Boil for 10 minutes, then drain the potato and discard the water.

2. In the slow cooker, combine the sweet potato, water, carrots, celery, onion, salt, and pepper and stir.

3. Cover and cook on low for 6 to 8 hours, or until the vegetables are tender.

4. Stir in the peas and cook on high for 10 minutes.

5. To serve, ladle into bowls and top each with 1 tablespoon of olive oil.

Ingredient Tip: To give this stew an Italian flair, add 1 teaspoon of dried Italian seasoning when you stir in the peas and serve the soup with some grated Parmesan or Romano cheese.

Per Serving Calories: 259; Total fat: 14g; Saturated fat: 2g; Sodium: 263mg; Phosphorus: 122mg; Potassium: 566mg; Carbohydrates: 19g; Fiber: 6g; Protein: 5g; Sugar: 8g

Spinach and Crab Soup

DIABETES-FRIENDLY, GLUTEN-FREE, HIGH PROTEIN

Serves 4 / Prep Time: 15 minutes / Cook Time: 10 minutes

This beautiful and zesty soup uses lump crab meat, fresh baby spinach, and Old Bay Seasoning, which is a classic spice mix used with seafood. If you can't find Old Bay, you can substitute ½ teaspoon of celery salt and ⅛ teaspoon each of cayenne pepper, nutmeg, paprika, and dry mustard. This soup is perfect for entertaining or for a cozy meal at home.

2 tablespoons extra-virgin olive oil

2 shallots, minced

8 ounces fresh lump crab meat, picked over

4 cups low-sodium vegetable broth

2 cups roughly chopped baby spinach leaves

½ teaspoon Old Bay Seasoning

⅛ teaspoon freshly ground black pepper

1. In a medium saucepan, heat the olive oil over medium heat. Cook the shallots for about 3 minutes, stirring, until tender.

2. Add the crab meat and cook for 1 minute. Add the vegetable broth and bring to a simmer. Reduce the heat to low.

3. Add the spinach leaves, Old Bay Seasoning mix, and pepper. Simmer until the spinach is wilted and the soup is hot. Serve.

Ingredient Tip: You could use other greens in place of the spinach. Try baby arugula leaves, frisée, or kale that has been torn into pieces.

Per Serving Calories: 138; Total fat: 7g; Saturated fat: 1g; Sodium: 408mg; Phosphorus: 160mg; Potassium: 345mg; Carbohydrates: 6g; Fiber: 1g; Protein: 12g; Sugar: 3g

Curried Lentil Soup

DIABETES-FRIENDLY, GLUTEN-FREE, HIGH FIBER, MEDIUM PROTEIN, VEGAN

Serves 4 / Prep Time: 15 minutes / Cook Time: 30 minutes

Lentils are an excellent staple on the renal diet because they're filled with fiber and plant protein. Boiling them in water for 10 minutes before they are cooked in the soup cuts the potassium level by about 50 percent. If you're limiting your protein intake, lentils are a great option; however, avoid combining them with other protein sources such as dairy, meat, or other kinds of legumes. Combining multiple protein sources at a time will result in a meal that is too high in protein.

½ cup green lentils, sorted

2 tablespoons extra-virgin olive oil

1 yellow onion, chopped

1 tablespoon curry powder

4 cups low-sodium vegetable broth

2 large carrots, peeled and sliced

⅛ teaspoon salt

⅛ teaspoon freshly ground
    black pepper

1. In a medium saucepan, combine the lentils and the amount of water on the lentil package's instructions. Bring to a boil over medium heat. Reduce the heat to low and simmer for 10 minutes. Drain well, discarding the water.

2. In a large saucepan, heat the olive oil over medium heat. Add the onion and curry powder and cook for about 3 minutes, stirring until the onion is tender.

3. Add the lentils, broth, carrots, salt, and pepper and bring to a simmer. Simmer for 20 minutes or until the carrots and lentils are tender. Serve.

Increase Protein Tip: To make this a high-protein recipe, top each serving with 2 tablespoons of nonfat plain Greek yogurt. The protein content will increase to 11g per serving.

Per Serving Calories: 186; Total fat: 8g; Saturated fat: 1g; Sodium: 240mg; Phosphorus: 101mg; Potassium: 379mg; Carbohydrates: 24g; Fiber: 5g; Protein: 7g; Sugar: 5g

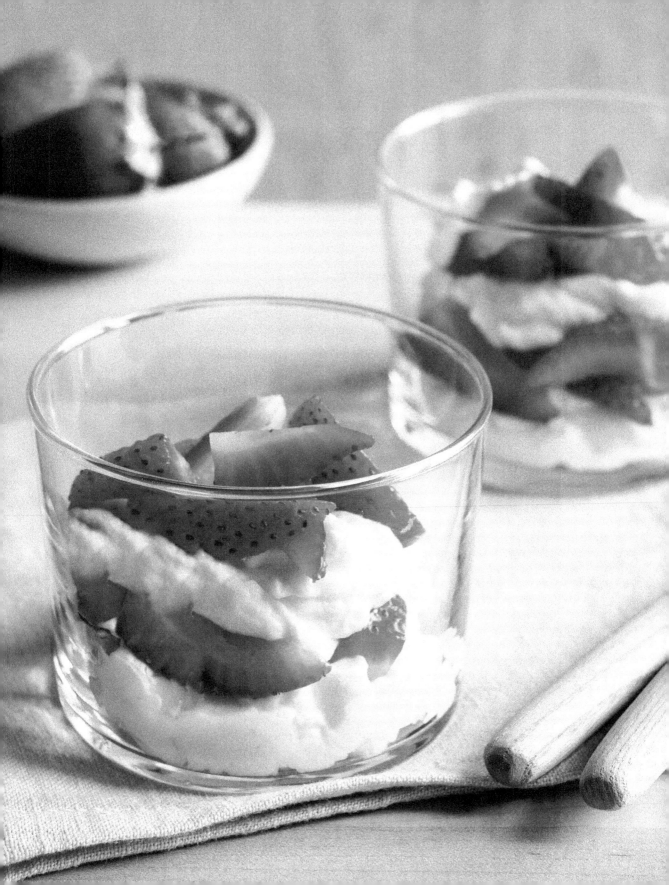

Desserts

⇐No-Cook Velvety Cheesecake Parfaits, page 121

Peach Pecan Crisp

HIGH FIBER, LOW PROTEIN, VEGETARIAN

Serves 8 / Prep Time: 20 minutes / Cook Time: 30 minutes

You may have had apple crisp made with a flour streusel on top. But did you know you don't have to use flour for a crisp and tender streusel? This recipe combines whole oats with ground oats for a fabulous texture and an extra helping of fiber. Peaches are swapped for apples, and the finished product is simply delicious!

Olive oil cooking spray

1½ cups rolled oats, divided

8 tablespoons brown sugar, divided

⅓ cup chopped pecans

¼ cup butter, melted

4 peaches, peeled and sliced

1. Preheat the oven to 350°F. Spray a 9-inch square baking dish with cooking spray and set aside.

2. In a large bowl, pour 1¼ cups of oats and set aside.

3. In a food processor, place the remaining ¼ cup of oats and process until fine. Add to the rolled oats and mix.

4. Add 6 tablespoons of brown sugar, the pecans, and the butter to the oat mixture and mix until crumbly.

5. Combine the peaches and remaining 2 tablespoons of brown sugar in the prepared baking dish. Top with the oat mixture.

6. Bake for 25 to 30 minutes, or until the peaches are bubbling and the streusel is golden brown. Let cool for 20 minutes, then serve.

Ingredient Tip: Simple swaps can make this recipe vegan and gluten-free. Replacing the butter with vegan butter and the oats with gluten-free oats is all that is needed.

Per Serving Calories: 203; Total fat: 10g; Saturated fat: 4g; Sodium: 49mg; Phosphorus: 92mg; Potassium: 230mg; Carbohydrates: 27g; Fiber: 3g; Protein: 3g; Sugar: 15g

Peanut Butter Chocolate Fudge

DIABETES-FRIENDLY, GLUTEN-FREE, HIGH FIBER, LOW PROTEIN, VEGETARIAN

Makes 18 pieces / Prep Time: 5 minutes / Cook Time: 5 minutes

Fudge is the ultimate indulgence. This combination of dark chocolate chips and peanut butter produces the most wonderful candy with hardly any effort. The phosphorus in this recipe is entirely from plant sources, which means much of it will not be absorbed in your body. Dark chocolate is rich in antioxidants and fiber.

1 (12-ounce) package 60 percent (or higher) cacao chocolate chips

⅓ cup peanut butter

1 tablespoon butter

1. Line an 8-inch square baking dish with parchment paper and set aside.
2. In a medium microwave-safe bowl, combine the chocolate chips, peanut butter, and butter. Microwave on 70 percent power for 1 minute; remove and stir. Continue microwaving for 30-second intervals, stirring each time, until the mixture is melted and smooth.
3. Pour into the prepared pan and smooth the top.
4. Refrigerate the fudge for 1 hour. Store for up to 5 days, covered, at room temperature.

Appliance Tip: You can make this recipe on the stovetop. Just combine the ingredients in a medium-size heavy saucepan and melt over low heat, stirring frequently, until the mixture is melted and smooth.

Per Serving (1 piece) Calories: 143; Total fat: 10g; Saturated fat: 5g; Sodium: 27mg; Phosphorus: 65mg; Potassium: 134mg; Carbohydrates: 11g; Fiber: 2g; Protein: 2g; Sugar: 7g

Rice Pudding with Raspberry Sauce

GLUTEN-FREE, HIGH FIBER, LOW PROTEIN, VEGETARIAN

Serves 6 / Prep Time: 5 minutes / Cook Time: 3 hours

Rice pudding is one of the easiest desserts to make. This one has a twist; some cream cheese is stirred in at the end of the cooking time to make the pudding rich and decadent. A simple raspberry sauce is the perfect finishing touch.

2 cups unsweetened vanilla
  almond milk
½ cup white rice
⅓ cup sugar
⅛ teaspoon salt

2 ounces cream cheese, at
  room temperature
1 (10-ounce) bag frozen
  raspberries, thawed

1. In a 3-quart slow cooker, combine the almond milk, rice, sugar, and salt. Cover and cook on low for 2 hours. Cooking on high will make the rice cook unevenly.

2. Stir the pudding, cover again, and cook for another 1 to 1½ hours or until the rice is very tender.

3. Stir in the cream cheese until melted.

4. Transfer to a bowl and place in the refrigerator until the rice pudding is chilled.

5. In a blender or food processor, place the raspberries and blend until smooth. Pour into a bowl.

6. You can serve the rice pudding after it's cooled, about 30 minutes. If you serve it cold, stir it again and serve with the raspberry sauce. Cover and store the raspberry sauce up to 3 days in the fridge.

Ingredient Tip: Feel free to try this rice pudding with brown rice. The cook time will change from 3 hours to 4 hours.

Per Serving Calories: 169; Total fat: 5g; Saturated fat: 2g; Sodium: 140mg; Phosphorus: 50mg; Potassium: 171mg; Carbohydrates: 30g; Fiber: 2g; Protein: 3g; Sugar: 15g

No-Cook Velvety Cheesecake Parfaits

GLUTEN-FREE, MEDIUM PROTEIN, VEGETARIAN

Serves 4 / Prep Time: 20 minutes

This cheesecake parfait recipe is perfect for summertime when you want to enjoy homemade dessert without having to turn on the oven. A no-bake cheesecake mixture is layered with strawberries in parfait glasses. If berries are not typically part of your diet, now is the time to change that! Not only are berries super nutritious, they are also low-potassium. Create a new version of this recipe by replacing strawberries with blueberries, blackberries, raspberries, or a combination!

---

1 (8-ounce) package cream cheese, at room temperature

⅓ cup powdered sugar

½ cup heavy cream

1 teaspoon vanilla extract

1½ cups chopped strawberries

---

1. In a medium bowl using a hand mixer on medium, beat the cream cheese and the powdered sugar until soft and well-blended.

2. In a small bowl using the mixer on high, beat the cream and vanilla for 4 to 6 minutes, until soft peaks form. Fold the whipped cream into the cream cheese mixture.

3. Into glasses, layer the cream cheese mixture with the strawberries. For an extra-fancy presentation, use parfait or stemmed glasses. Cover and chill for 2 to 3 hours before serving.

Diabetes Tip: To make this recipe diabetes-friendly, omit the powdered sugar and replace with ⅓ cup plus 2 tablespoons of powdered erythritol. The carbohydrate content will decrease to 9g.

Per Serving Calories: 359; Total fat: 30g; Saturated fat: 18g; Sodium: 187mg; Phosphorus: 92mg; Potassium: 192mg; Carbohydrates: 18g; Fiber: 1g; Protein: 5g; Sugar: 16g

Peanut Butter Coconut Bars

HIGH FIBER, LOW PROTEIN, VEGETARIAN

Makes 25 bars / Prep Time: 10 minutes / Cook Time: 5 minutes, plus 3 hours to set

This no-bake bar recipe is perfect when you want something sweet but don't feel like baking. Both creamy and crunchy peanut butter would work in this recipe; choose whichever you prefer. Many people are under the false impression that peanut butter is not allowed on the renal diet. This is an old-fashioned idea, based on the concern that peanut butter is high in phosphorus. While peanut butter does have phosphorus, it's also high in phytic acid, which prevents a significant amount of the phosphorus from being absorbed.

1¼ cups peanut butter, divided

½ cup honey

1¼ cups graham cracker crumbs

1 cup unsweetened shredded
   coconut flakes

1 cup 60 percent cacao
   chocolate chips

1. In a large saucepan, combine 1 cup of peanut butter and the honey over medium heat. Melt, stirring frequently.

2. Add the graham cracker crumbs and coconut and stir until combined. Press into an 8-inch square pan.

3. In a small microwave-safe bowl, combine the remaining ¼ cup of peanut butter and the chocolate chips. Microwave on high for 30 seconds; remove and stir. Continue microwaving for 30-second intervals, stirring after each interval, until the mixture is smooth.

4. Pour over the bars and let stand for 3 hours to cool and set.

5. When cool, cut into 5 strips and then cut those strips into 5.

Ingredient Tip: This recipe would also work with other nut and seed butters such as almond butter and sunflower seed butter.

Per Serving (1 bar) Calories: 179; Total fat: 12g; Saturated fat: 5g; Sodium: 79mg; Phosphorus: 77mg; Potassium: 141mg; Carbohydrates: 16g; Fiber: 2g; Protein: 4g; Sugar: 11g

Mixed Berry Fruit Salad

DIABETES-FRIENDLY, GLUTEN-FREE, HIGH FIBER, LOW PROTEIN, VEGETARIAN

Serves 4 / Prep Time: 20 minutes

For people with diabetes, eating fruit may lead to a blood sugar level spike. This is especially the case for tropical fruits such as pineapple and mango. This fruit salad avoids the high-sugar fruits, focusing instead on berries—the fruit least likely to spike blood sugar. Sour cream, a fat source that is essentially sugar-free, will help slow down the digestion of the berries, which also helps control blood sugar. Use the best berries you can find for this simple end to the meal.

1½ cups raspberries, divided

1½ cups sliced strawberries

1 cup blackberries

⅓ cup sour cream

1 tablespoon chopped fresh
  mint leaves

---

1. In a medium bowl, combine 1¼ cups of raspberries with the strawberries and blackberries and mix gently.

2. In a small bowl, place the remaining ¼ cup of raspberries and crush with a fork. Stir in the sour cream and mint leaves.

3. Divide into serving cups, top with the sour cream mixture, and serve.

Make It Easier Tip: Instead of the chopped fresh mint leaves, you can add a few drops of mint extract to the sour cream. It's easy to go overboard, so add the extract just a drop at a time and taste as you go.

Per Serving Calories: 95; Total fat: 4g; Saturated fat: 2g; Sodium: 7mg; Phosphorus: 49mg; Potassium: 239mg; Carbohydrates: 14g; Fiber: 6g; Protein: 2g; Sugar: 7g

Peach-Filled Meringue

GLUTEN-FREE, HIGH FIBER, LOW PROTEIN, VEGETARIAN

Serves 6 / Prep Time: 40 minutes / Cook Time: 1 hour

These individual little meringues are the perfect choice for dessert at a dinner party or barbecue. The meringues have to be made ahead of time, but last-minute assembly is a snap. Powdered sugar is used instead of granulated sugar because it dissolves more easily and also contains cornstarch, which helps keep the meringue soft in the middle. Because this recipe uses egg whites without any egg yolks, it contains very little phosphorus. The sugar content is high, however, so be sure to limit this treat to special occasions.

4 large egg whites

1 cup powdered sugar

2 teaspoons freshly squeezed
  lemon juice, divided

½ cup heavy whipping cream

4 fresh peaches, peeled
  and chopped

1. Preheat the oven to 350°F. Line a baking sheet with parchment paper and set aside.

2. The egg whites should be at room temperature, so let them stand for 20 minutes after you have separated them.

3. Once the egg whites are at room temperature, place them into a bowl and using a hand mixer on high, beat for about 3 minutes, until peaks begin to form. Beat in the powdered sugar 2 tablespoons at a time for about 3 to 5 minutes longer.

4. Fold in 1 teaspoon of lemon juice.

5. To keep the parchment paper from sliding off the baking sheet, dab a bit of the meringue on the bottom side and put back onto the baking sheet.

6. Form 6 small circles of the meringue, about 4 inches across and 1 inch thick, on the parchment paper.

7. Place in the oven and reduce the heat immediately to 300°F. Bake for 1 hour, then turn off the heat, open the oven door slightly, and let the meringues cool.

8. In a medium bowl and using a hand mixer on high, beat the cream for 4 to 6 minutes, until soft peaks form. Fold in the remaining 1 teaspoon of lemon juice and the peaches.

9. Turn the little meringues over and top with the cream mixture. Cover and refrigerate for 2 to 3 hours, then serve.

Ingredient Tip: It's easier to separate egg whites from the yolks while the egg is cold. Crack the egg and gently pry the two halves of the shell open. Over a small bowl, rock the yolk from one shell to the other until all the egg white is in the bowl. Transfer the white to a large bowl for beating and repeat. Let stand for at least 20 minutes after separating to reach room temperature.

Per Serving Calories: 196; Total fat: 7g; Saturated fat: 5g; Sodium: 43mg; Phosphorus: 34mg; Potassium: 247mg; Carbohydrates: 30g; Fiber: 2g; Protein: 4g; Sugar: 29g

Filo Apple Hand Pies

MEDIUM PROTEIN, VEGETARIAN

Serves 8 / Prep Time: 25 minutes / Cook Time: 25 minutes

No fork, no plate, no problem! Just pick up and enjoy one of these cute little apple-filled pastry pockets. One hand pie is the perfect portion, and the leftover pies can be frozen for another time. They are fun and easy to make. As long as you keep the filo stack covered with a damp (not wet) towel as you work, and handle the sheets gently, you'll have success.

---

1 medium Granny Smith apple,
   peeled and chopped
¼ cup sugar

6 tablespoons butter, divided
1 teaspoon vanilla extract
8 (9-by-14-inch) filo sheets, thawed

---

1. In a medium saucepan, combine the apples, sugar, and 2 tablespoons of butter. Bring to a simmer over medium heat, then reduce heat to low and simmer for 5 to 7 minutes or until the apples are tender. Transfer to a bowl and place in the freezer to cool for 30 minutes.

2. Remove the apple mixture from the freezer, add the vanilla, and stir.

3. Preheat the oven to 350°F.

4. In a small saucepan, melt the remaining 4 tablespoons of butter and pour into a small bowl.

5. Place one of the filo sheets on the work surface and brush with a bit of the butter. Layer one more sheet onto the first sheet.

6. Fold the filo stack in half to make a 4½-by-14-inch rectangle. Put 2 to 3 tablespoons of the apple mixture on the end of the strip. Fold the bottom right corner up to the left side so the bottom becomes the left side, then fold straight. Bring the bottom left corner up to the right side and fold straight. Seal the pastry with a bit of butter and place on a baking sheet.

7. Repeat with the remaining filo, butter, and apple filling. Brush all the pastries with the remaining butter.

8. Bake for 15 to 20 minutes or until the filo is crisp and golden brown. Remove to a cooling rack to cool and set aside.

Make It Easier Tip: You can assemble these little pies up to 8 hours ahead of time and then put them in the fridge. When you're ready, bake as directed, adding a few minutes of baking time for the cold pies.

Ingredient Tip: You can refreeze filo dough. Just wrap it in the original wrapping, put it back into the box, seal the box with tape, and freeze. You can also freeze the little pies once they are completely cool.

Per Serving (1 hand pie) Calories: 236; Total fat: 9g; Saturated fat: 5g; Sodium: 168mg; Phosphorus: 39mg; Potassium: 59mg; Carbohydrates: 35g; Fiber: 1g; Protein: 4g; Sugar: 9g

Watermelon Mint Granita

GLUTEN-FREE, LOW PROTEIN, VEGAN

Serves 4 / Prep Time: 15 minutes, plus 2 hours to chill

What could be more refreshing than a blend of watermelon, lemons, and mint leaves? Blend them together and freeze, and you have the perfect treat in the heat. A granita is simply juice that has been frozen. To serve, the frozen juice is scraped with a fork into tiny pieces and scooped into a stemmed glass. To increase the healthiness of this dessert, experiment with using less sugar. Just like salt, you can train your taste buds to desire less!

4 cups watermelon cubes, seeded
¼ cup sugar
2 tablespoons freshly squeezed
   lemon juice

2 tablespoons minced fresh
   mint leaves

1. In a blender or food processor, combine the watermelon, sugar, lemon juice, and mint and blend until smooth.

2. Pour the mixture into a 9-inch square pan. Freeze for 2 hours, stirring the mixture once during freezing time.

3. To serve, scrape up some of the granita with a fork and spoon lightly into glasses.

Make It Easier Tip: Buy seedless watermelon and you won't have to remove the seeds. There are still seeds in seedless watermelon, but they are so small and tender you can eat them.

Per Serving Calories: 81; Total fat: 0g; Saturated fat: 0g; Sodium: 1mg; Phosphorus: 12mg; Potassium: 123mg; Carbohydrates: 21g; Fiber: 0g; Protein: 1g; Sugar: 19g

Peanut Butter Mug Cake

GLUTEN-FREE, HIGH FIBER, HIGH PROTEIN, VEGETARIAN

Serves 1 / Prep Time: 5 minutes / Cook Time: 2 minutes

When you feel like a sweet treat but don't feel like going through all the steps of baking a cake, a mug cake is the answer. A mug cake is a small cake that is made, well, in a coffee mug. This recipe is also a great choice for when you don't have many ingredients on hand. It makes one cake and is ready in about 5 minutes.

3 tablespoons gluten-free
   flour blend

2 tablespoons peanut butter

2 tablespoons almond milk

4 teaspoons brown sugar

¼ teaspoon Low-Phosphorus
   Baking Powder (page 144)

1. In an 8-ounce microwave-safe mug, combine the flour blend, peanut butter, almond milk, brown sugar, and baking powder and stir until combined.

2. Microwave on high for 45 to 60 seconds or until the cake springs back when lightly touched with a finger. If the cake isn't done, microwave for 10-second intervals until it does spring back.

3. Let cool for 3 to 4 minutes and eat.

Ingredient Tip: Stir in 1 tablespoon of chocolate chips before cooking this little cake for a Chocolate Peanut Butter Mug Cake.

Per Serving (1 cake) Calories: 482; Total fat: 28g; Saturated fat: 7g; Sodium: 230mg; Phosphorus: 217mg; Potassium: 384mg; Carbohydrates: 48g; Fiber: 3g; Protein: 14g; Sugar: 24g

Almond-Cranberry Cookies

GLUTEN-FREE, HIGH FIBER, LOW PROTEIN, VEGETARIAN

Makes 16 cookies / Prep Time: 15 minutes / Cook Time: 15 minutes

When entertaining guests, it's a good idea to offer at least one gluten-free dessert option. These little cookies are a perfect choice with the combination of tart and sweetness but not too much of either. Almond butter acts as the structure for these cookies along with the egg. Don't worry about whether the jar of almond butter says "salted" or "unsalted," as the amount of sodium in the salted version is negligible.

¾ cup brown sugar	½ teaspoon vanilla extract
1 large egg	⅛ teaspoon salt
1 cup almond butter	½ cup dried cranberries

1. Preheat the oven to 350°F. Line a baking sheet with parchment paper and set aside.

2. In a medium bowl, mix the brown sugar and egg until smooth.

3. Add the almond butter, vanilla, and salt and beat until a soft dough forms. Work in the cranberries.

4. Spoon onto the prepared baking sheet by generous tablespoons.

5. Bake for 13 to 17 minutes or until the cookies are lightly browned on the edges. Let cool on the baking sheet for 2 minutes, then carefully transfer to a cooling rack.

6. Store covered at room temperature for up to 3 days.

Ingredient Tip: You can make your own almond butter; it just takes 2 cups of whole unsalted roasted almonds and a little cinnamon or honey if you'd like. Place the almonds into a high-speed blender or a food processor and puree on high. It will take some time to reach almond butter consistency; just keep pureeing and scraping down the sides of the blender or food processor. Store in a covered container in the fridge for up to 2 weeks.

Per Serving (1 cookie) Calories: 156; Total fat: 9g; Saturated fat: 1g; Sodium: 62mg; Phosphorus: 86mg; Potassium: 137mg; Carbohydrates: 17g; Fiber: 2g; Protein: 4g; Sugar: 14g

Dark Chocolate Mousse

GLUTEN-FREE, HIGH FIBER, MEDIUM PROTEIN, VEGETARIAN

Serves 10 / Prep Time: 10 minutes, plus 1 hour to chill / Cook Time: 10 minutes

Chocolate mousse is so creamy and delicious. This recipe has peanut butter that helps mellow the dark chocolate's bitterness and adds wonderful smoothness. When purchasing dark chocolate chips, look for a brand with the highest percentage of cocoa that you can find. The higher the percentage, the more nutrient dense the chocolate is.

2 cups dark chocolate chips

7 tablespoons peanut butter, divided

1 cup heavy whipping cream, divided

2 teaspoons powdered sugar

½ teaspoon vanilla extract

1. In a large bowl, combine the chocolate chips and 6 tablespoons of peanut butter.

2. In a medium saucepan, heat ¾ cup of cream over medium heat until steam rises from the surface; don't let the cream boil.

3. Add the cream all at once to the chocolate peanut butter mixture and stir until the chocolate melts and the mixture is smooth.

4. Cover and refrigerate for 1 hour until firm.

5. Remove the chocolate mixture from the fridge and, using a hand mixer on medium high, beat for 3 to 4 minutes, until it's fluffy. Do not overbeat. Spoon into 6 dessert cups.

6. In a small bowl using a mixer on high, beat the remaining ¼ cup of cream, remaining 1 tablespoon of peanut butter, powdered sugar, and vanilla until stiff. Dollop this mixture on top of the cups and serve.

Diabetes-Friendly Tip: If you use sugar-free dark chocolate chips for this recipe, the carbohydrate content will decrease to 14g and the sugar content to 2g per serving.

Per Serving Calories: 362; Total fat: 28g; Saturated fat: 15g; Sodium: 58mg; Phosphorus: 146mg; Potassium: 292mg; Carbohydrates: 23g; Fiber: 3g; Protein: 5g; Sugar: 16g

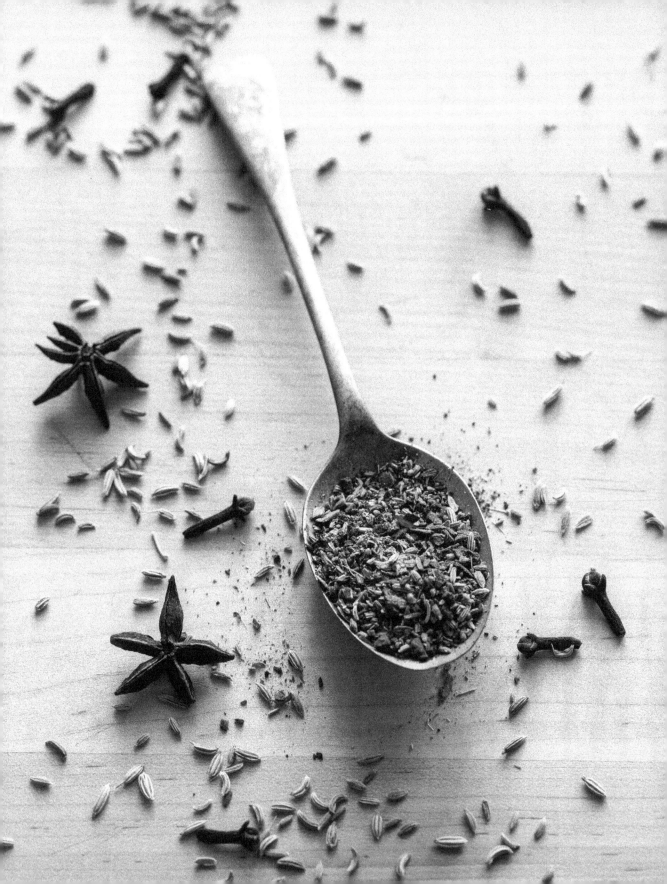

CHAPTER 8

Broths, Condiments, and Seasoning Mixes

⇐ *Five-Spice Blend, page 147*

Homemade Pizza Crust

MEDIUM PROTEIN, HIGH FIBER, VEGAN

Makes 2 pizza crusts (8 slices per crust) / Prep Time: 20 minutes,
plus 1 hour to proof / Cook Time: 25 minutes

It's easy to create your own pizza with this simple recipe that makes two 12-inch crusts. Cornmeal adds crunch, and whole-wheat flour makes this crust high in fiber. Just top the crust with your choice of toppings, such as your favorite veggies and a pesto sauce, and bake for a delicious pizza everyone will enjoy.

1 cup all-purpose flour
1 cup whole-wheat flour
½ cup yellow cornmeal
1 (0.25 ounce) package active
   dry yeast

¼ teaspoon salt
1 cup warm water
2 tablespoons extra-virgin olive oil,
   plus more for oiling the bowl

1. In a large bowl, combine the flours, cornmeal, yeast, and salt and mix well.

2. Add the water and olive oil and mix until a firm dough forms.

3. Place the dough on a lightly floured surface and knead for 5 to 7 minutes or until the dough is smooth. To knead, press the dough away from you and double it onto itself. Repeat this process, turning the dough as you work, until it's smooth.

4. Grease a large bowl with a bit of olive oil and add the dough. Turn the dough over in the bowl to grease the dough's top layer. Cover with a towel and let stand at room temperature until the dough rises and is doubled in bulk, about an hour.

5. After an hour, remove the dough and place it back on lightly floured surface. Punch down with your fist, divide in half, and form each half into a 5-inch disc. At this point you can put the dough into freezer bags, label, seal, and freeze up to 5 months. To thaw, let stand overnight in the fridge.

6. Spray two 12-inch pizza pans with nonstick baking spray and add one dough ball to each. Using a rolling pin, roll the dough out until the pan is evenly covered with it.

7. Preheat the oven to 400°F.

8. Top the dough with desired toppings and bake for 20 to 25 minutes or until the crust is golden brown, and the cheese (if using) is melted and golden brown in spots. Cut into wedges to serve.

Cooking Tip: The water temperature used to dissolve yeast is crucial. It will kill the yeast if it's too hot, but the yeast won't activate if it's too cold. The water should feel warm to the touch, but not hot enough to hurt, which is about 120°F if you're using a thermometer.

Per Serving (2 slices) Calories: 168; Total fat: 4g; Saturated fat: 1g; Sodium: 151mg; Phosphorus: 94mg; Potassium: 102mg; Carbohydrates: 29g; Fiber: 3g; Protein: 5g; Sugar: 0g

Romesco Sauce

Makes 2 cups / Prep Time: 5 minutes / Cook Time: 5 minutes

Romesco sauce is usually made with tomatoes, roasted red bell peppers, almonds, and garlic. This recipe omits the tomatoes completely to help reduce the phosphorus and potassium content. It's smooth and delicious served over grilled fish or chicken, drizzled over roasted vegetables, or used as a pizza or pasta sauce. You can even use it as an appetizer dip.

---

1 (16-ounce) jar roasted red
   peppers, drained
¼ cup slivered almonds
2 tablespoons extra-virgin olive oil
2 tablespoons freshly squeezed
   lemon juice

1 garlic clove, peeled
½ teaspoon paprika
Pinch salt

In a food processor or blender, combine the red peppers, almonds, olive oil, lemon juice, garlic, paprika, and salt. Process or blend until the mixture is smooth. Store covered in the fridge up to 5 days.

Per serving (2 tablespoons) Calories: 67; Total fat: 5g; Saturated fat: 1g; Sodium: 245mg; Phosphorus: 32mg; Potassium: 155mg; Carbohydrates: 4g; Fiber: 1g; Protein: 1g; Sugar: 3g

Vegetable Broth

DIABETES-FRIENDLY, GLUTEN-FREE, LOW PROTEIN, VEGAN

Makes 5 cups / Prep Time: 20 minutes / Cook Time: 4 hours

Vegetable broth is an essential ingredient in many of these recipes. Making your own is easy and adds much more flavor than canned or boxed broths, which often contain excessive sodium amounts. When you have CKD and are following a low-protein diet, vegetable broth is a tasty, low-protein substitute for chicken or beef broth.

1 tablespoon extra-virgin olive oil
1 unpeeled onion, sliced
2 unpeeled carrots, sliced
2 celery stalks, sliced
2 unpeeled garlic cloves, crushed

6 cups water
1 teaspoon dried basil leaves
½ teaspoon salt
⅛ teaspoon freshly ground
   black pepper

1. In a large saucepan, heat the olive oil over medium-high heat.
2. Add the onion, carrots, celery, and garlic and brown for 5 minutes, stirring frequently.
3. Add the water, basil, salt, and pepper and bring to a boil.
4. Reduce the heat to medium low and simmer for 3 to 4 hours, stirring occasionally. Skim off and discard any foam that rises to the surface.
5. Strain the broth into a colander set over a bowl. Discard the solids.
6. Refrigerate the broth. When it's cold, remove the fat that rises to the top. You can freeze this broth in 1-cup freezer-safe containers to use in recipes.

Ingredient Tip: You can use any vegetables you'd like in this recipe, but avoid potatoes and sweet potatoes because they make the broth cloudy. You can also use leftover veggie scraps to make this since you're not eating the veggies; you just need their flavor.

Per Serving (½ cup) Calories: 25; Total fat: 1g; Saturated fat: 0g; Sodium: 17mg; Phosphorus: 12 mg; Potassium: 88mg; Carbohydrates: 3g; Fiber: 1g; Protein: 0g; Sugar: 1g

Chicken Stock

DIABETES-FRIENDLY, GLUTEN-FREE, HIGH PROTEIN

Makes 8 cups / Prep Time: 15 minutes / Cook Time: 4 hours

Homemade chicken stock might seem like a big undertaking, but it's actually pretty easy to make. The onions, carrots, and garlic do not need any peeling, and the only seasonings added are salt, pepper, and a bay leaf. When making stock or broth, it's time that counts, not the number of ingredients you use.

4 bone-in, skin-on chicken thighs (about 1½ pounds)
2 unpeeled onions, sliced
2 unpeeled carrots, sliced
3 unpeeled garlic cloves
1 tablespoon extra-virgin olive oil

⅛ teaspoon salt
⅛ teaspoon freshly ground black pepper
8 cups water
1 bay leaf

1. Preheat the oven to 400°F.

2. On a rimmed baking sheet, combine the chicken, onions, carrots, and garlic. Drizzle with the olive oil, salt, and pepper and toss to coat.

3. Roast for 45 to 55 minutes or until the chicken reads 165°F and the juices run clear and the vegetables are lightly browned.

4. Remove the ingredients from the baking sheet. Remove the garlic from its skins, discarding the skins. Place the vegetables in a large saucepan. Set the chicken aside to cool for 15 minutes.

5. Remove the meat from the skin and bones. Discard the skin; reserve the meat for another use. You can freeze the meat for up to 3 months. Place the bones into the saucepan with the vegetables.

6. Add the water and bay leaf to the saucepan.

7. Bring to a boil over high heat, then reduce the heat to low and simmer for 3 to 4 hours or until the broth is golden brown.

8. Strain the stock into a colander set over a bowl. Discard the vegetables, bones, and bay leaf.

9. Refrigerate the broth. When it's cold, remove the fat that rises to the top. You can freeze this broth in 2-cup freezer-safe containers to use in recipes.

Reduce Protein Tip: To make this a medium-protein recipe, you can use two bone-in, skin-on chicken breasts. In step 3, roast instead for 20 to 25 minutes or until the chicken is done, then proceed with the recipe. The protein content will decrease to 6g per serving.

Per Serving (½ cup) Calories: 119; Total fat: 7g; Saturated fat: 2g; Sodium: 74mg; Phosphorus: 78mg; Potassium: 152mg; Carbohydrates: 2g; Fiber: 0g; Protein: 12g; Sugar: 1g

Grainy Mustard

Makes about ½ cup / Prep Time: 15 minutes

If you love the sharp and pungent flavor that mustard brings to recipes, you'll really appreciate the taste of homemade grainy mustard. Making your own mustard is quick and easy. While most store-bought mustards tend to contain low to moderate amounts of sodium, this recipe creates a mustard that is extremely low in sodium. Only a small amount of salt is used, with additional flavors coming from lemon juice, apple cider vinegar, and turmeric.

¼ cup dry mustard

¼ cup mustard seeds

¼ cup apple cider vinegar

3 tablespoons water

2 tablespoons freshly squeezed lemon juice

½ teaspoon ground turmeric

⅛ teaspoon salt

1. In a jar with a tight-fitting lid, combine the mustard, mustard seeds, vinegar, water, lemon juice, turmeric, and salt and stir to combine.

2. Refrigerate the mustard for 5 days, stirring once a day and adding a bit more water every day, as the mustard will thicken as it stands. It should look like the mustard you buy from the store.

3. After 5 days, the mustard is ready to use. Refrigerate in a covered container up to 2 weeks.

Per Serving (1 teaspoon) Calories: 22; Total fat: 2g; Saturated fat: 1g; Sodium: 13mg; Phosphorus: 9mg; Potassium: 13mg; Carbohydrates: 1g; Fiber: 0g; Protein: 1g; Sugar: 0g

Salsa Verde

DIABETES-FRIENDLY, GLUTEN-FREE, LOW PROTEIN, VEGAN

Makes 2 cups / Prep Time: 20 minutes / Cook Time: 15 minutes

Salsa verde simply means "green salsa"; in this case, it's a cooked sauce. It's a combination of tomatillos (a mandarin orange–size green tomato), jalapeño peppers, and lime juice that makes a spicy, refreshing salsa you can use on just about anything, from fish to a salad to an appetizer. If you don't have access to fresh tomatillos, canned will work just fine.

---

2 cups halved tomatillos or
  1 (11-ounce) can tomatillos,
  drained
3 scallions, both green and white
  parts, chopped
1 jalapeño pepper, chopped

2 tablespoons extra-virgin olive oil
⅓ cup cilantro leaves
2 tablespoons freshly squeezed
  lime juice
⅛ teaspoon salt

---

1. Preheat the oven to 400°F.
2. On a rimmed baking sheet, combine the tomatillos, scallions, and jalapeño pepper.
3. Drizzle with the olive oil and toss to coat.
4. Roast the vegetables for 12 to 17 minutes or until the tomatillos are soft and light golden brown around the edges.
5. In a blender or food processor, combine the roasted vegetables with the cilantro, lime juice, and salt. Blend until smooth.
6. Store the salsa verde in a covered container in the fridge up to 3 days or freeze up to 3 months.

Ingredient Tip: You can make this salsa as mild or as spicy as you'd like. Omit the jalapeño pepper for a milder version or use serrano peppers for more heat.

Per Serving (2 tablespoons) Calories: 22; Total fat: 2g; Saturated fat: 0g; Sodium: 20mg; Phosphorus: 8mg; Potassium: 55mg; Carbohydrates: 1g; Fiber: 0g; Protein: 0g; Sugar: 1g

Grape Salsa

Makes 2 cups / Prep Time: 15 minutes

Salsa is usually made with tomatoes and other vegetables, but this dish is delicious when made with fruit. This recipe uses grapes but would also work well with peaches. This is the perfect topping to serve at a summer barbecue or picnic. Try it as a condiment with your meal or serve it as an appetizer with unsalted tortilla chips. This recipe is also great for topping grilled fish or chicken.

1 cup coarsely chopped red grapes
1 cup coarsely chopped
   green grapes
½ cup chopped red onion
2 tablespoons freshly squeezed
   lime juice

1 tablespoon honey
⅛ teaspoon salt
¼ teaspoon freshly ground
   black pepper

1. In a medium bowl, combine the grapes, onion, lime juice, honey, salt, and pepper and mix gently.
2. Cover and chill for 1 to 2 hours before serving or serve immediately.

Ingredient Tip: You could substitute the red onions for scallions or minced shallots if you want a milder flavor. If you like your salsa hotter, add some minced jalapeños or dried red pepper flakes.

Per Serving (⅓ cup) Calories: 51; Total fat: 0g; Saturated fat: 0g; Sodium: 53 mg; Phosphorus: 14mg; Potassium: 121mg; Carbohydrates: 14g; Fiber: 1g; Protein: 1g; Sugar: 11g

Apple and Brown Sugar Chutney

GLUTEN-FREE, LOW PROTEIN, VEGAN

Makes 2 cups / Prep Time: 15 minutes / Cook Time: 1 hour

Chutney is simply a mixture of fruits and spices, cooked together until it forms a texture similar to jam. This recipe is delicious served with broiled or grilled fish or chicken, or as a dip for apple wedges.

3 Granny Smith apples, peeled
  and chopped
1 onion, chopped
1 cup water
½ cup golden raisins

⅓ cup brown sugar
2 teaspoons curry powder
⅛ teaspoon salt
⅛ teaspoon freshly ground
  black pepper

1. In a medium saucepan, combine the apples, onion, water, raisins, brown sugar, curry powder, salt, and pepper and bring to a boil over medium-high heat.

2. Reduce the heat to low and simmer, stirring occasionally, for 45 to 55 minutes or until the mixture has thickened and the apples are very tender.

3. Cool, then decant into jars or containers. Store covered in the fridge up to 2 weeks.

Per Serving (1 tablespoon) Calories: 27; Total fat: 0g; Saturated fat: 0g; Sodium: 11 mg; Phosphorus: 6mg; Potassium: 48mg; Carbohydrates: 7g; Fiber: 1 g; Protein: 0g; Sugar: 6g

Low-Phosphorus Baking Powder

DIABETES-FRIENDLY, GLUTEN-FREE, LOW PROTEIN, VEGAN

Makes 10 tablespoons / Prep Time: 20 minutes

Baking powder is very high in phosphorus. Luckily, it's easy to make a low-phosphorus version using just three ingredients. Baking powder's magic comes from the combination of alkaline and acidic components. When combined with liquid, they produce carbon dioxide, which makes baked goods rise. Since this ingredient is usually used in small amounts to make several servings of a baked good, the amount of potassium per serving of baked goods will be very low.

6 tablespoons cream of tartar

3 tablespoons baking soda

1 tablespoon cornstarch

1. In a small bowl, combine the cream of tartar, baking soda, and cornstarch and whisk to combine.

2. Press the mixture through a fine sieve to remove any lumps.

3. Store in an airtight container at room temperature and use in baking recipes.

Ingredient Tip: Most commercial baking powder is double-acting, which means it produces carbon dioxide when it gets wet and again in the heat of the oven. In single-acting baking powder like this one, the carbon dioxide is only produced when liquid is introduced. To get the best results with this powder, make sure to put the batter or dough into the oven as quickly as possible.

Per Serving (1 teaspoon) Calories: 6; Total fat: 0g; Saturated fat: 0g; Sodium: 379mg; Phosphorus: 0mg; Potassium: 297mg; Carbohydrates: 1g; Fiber: 0g; Protein: 0g; Sugar: 0g

No-Salt Seasoning Blend

DIABETES-FRIENDLY, GLUTEN-FREE, LOW PROTEIN, VEGAN

Makes 2 tablespoons / Prep Time: 10 minutes

This recipe can be made from your favorite dried herbs and spices. Just keep to the general proportions in this recipe and keep trying until you find your favorite blend. You can add more than five herbs too; they don't really have any effect on the protein, phosphorus, or potassium in your diet.

2 teaspoons dried thyme leaves

2 teaspoons dried marjoram leaves

2 teaspoons dried basil leaves

1 teaspoon dried oregano leaves

½ teaspoon onion powder

¼ teaspoon freshly ground black pepper

In a small jar with a tight-fitting lid, combine the thyme, marjoram, basil, oregano, onion powder, and pepper. Cover and store at room temperature for up to 6 months.

Ingredient Tip: Other herbs you can use in this blend include savory (the herb), sage, dill weed, dried parsley, and tarragon. You can also add celery seed, dill seed, fennel seed, or ground ginger.

Per Serving (¼ teaspoon) Calories: 1; Total fat: 0g; Saturated fat: 0g; Sodium: 0mg; Phosphorus: 1mg; Potassium: 4mg; Carbohydrates: 0g; Fiber: 0g; Protein: 0g; Sugar: 0g

Classic Spice Blend

DIABETES-FRIENDLY, GLUTEN-FREE, LOW PROTEIN, VEGAN

Makes 2 tablespoons / Prep Time: 10 minutes

The flavor in commercial spice blends tends to be salt heavy, and this can detract from the quality of your cooking. It's easy to make your own blend of spices. This combination of spices is a great substitute for salt and can add flavor to salad dressings, vegetables, and plain chicken or fish. Keep it stored in a glass jar with an airtight lid at room temperature for up to a year.

1 tablespoon whole
   black peppercorns
2 teaspoons caraway seeds

2 teaspoons celery seeds
1 teaspoon dill seeds
1 teaspoon cumin seeds

In a spice blender or in a mortar and pestle, combine the peppercorns, caraway seeds, celery seeds, dill seeds, and cumin. Grind until the seeds are broken down and the mixture almost becomes a powder.

Ingredient Tip: You can substitute other seeds or spices for the ones called for in this recipe. Try grains of paradise (a seed that is similar to peppercorns and cloves), mustard seeds, sesame seeds, or star anise. Be sure to make a note of the changes you've made so you can duplicate it.

Per Serving (¼ teaspoon) Calories: 2; Total fat: 0g; Saturated fat: 0g; Sodium: 0mg; Phosphorus: 3mg; Potassium: 8mg; Carbohydrates: 0g; Fiber: 0g; Protein: 0g; Sugar: 0g

Five-Spice Blend

Makes 2 tablespoons / Prep Time: 5 minutes

Five-spice is a classic mixture used in Chinese and Asian cooking. You can purchase this mixture already ground but grinding it yourself from whole spices makes a much more flavorful seasoning blend.

4 whole star anise

2 teaspoons white peppercorns

1 tablespoon fennel seeds

8 whole cloves

½ cinnamon stick

In a spice grinder or food processor, combine the star anise, peppercorns, fennel, cloves, and cinnamon stick and pulse until the mixture is fine. Store in an airtight container at room temperature up to 2 months.

Appliance Tip: A spice grinder is like a mini food processor. You can also use a coffee grinder if you prefer to grind the beans yourself. Just be sure to clean the coffee grinder well after you make this spice blend unless you want to drink Five-Spice Coffee!

Per Serving (½ teaspoon) Calories: 23; Total fat: 1g; Saturated Fat: 0g; Sodium: 8mg; Phosphorus: 6mg; Potassium: 14mg; Carbohydrates: 3g; Fiber: 1g; Protein: 0g; Sugar: 1g

Ranch Salad Dressing

DIABETES-FRIENDLY, GLUTEN-FREE, LOW PROTEIN, VEGETARIAN

Makes 1 cup / Prep Time: 5 minutes

Making your own salad dressing helps you avoid the many unhealthy ingredients added to store-bought dressings, such as refined oils and excess sugar and salt. This dressing gets its creaminess from plain Greek yogurt. It's best to use whole-milk Greek yogurt in this recipe as the fat in the yogurt assists your body in absorbing the vitamins in the veggies. This dressing is also an excellent dip for raw vegetables.

1 cup plain whole-milk Greek yogurt
½ teaspoon dried thyme
½ teaspoon dried dill weed
½ teaspoon dried chives

⅛ teaspoon salt
⅛ teaspoon freshly ground
    black pepper

In a small bowl, whisk the Greek yogurt, thyme, dill, chives, salt, and pepper until smooth. Store covered in the fridge up to 1 week.

Ingredient Tip: You can substitute any type of dried herb in this recipe that you'd like. Try dried oregano, onion powder, or garlic powder. If you like a lemon flavor, try some freshly grated lemon zest.

Per Serving (2 tablespoons) Calories: 26; Total fat: 1g; Saturated fat: 1g; Sodium: 50mg; Phosphorus: 26mg; Potassium: 45mg; Carbohydrates: 1g; Fiber: 0g; Protein: 3g; Sugar: 1g

Italian Salad Dressing

DIABETES-FRIENDLY, GLUTEN-FREE, LOW PROTEIN, VEGETARIAN

Makes 1 cup / Prep Time: 10 minutes

Italian salad dressing is a classic oil-and-vinegar dressing, but it's best made with white wine vinegar. You must use extra-virgin olive oil in this recipe because the flavor of the oil is so prominent. The use of olive oil in this recipe makes it a much healthier alternative to most of the salad dressings that line the shelves, as they tend to use cheaper and less healthy oils such as soybean oil. Make sure to shake this salad dressing before serving to emulsify the oil and vinegar again.

¾ cup extra-virgin olive oil

¼ cup white wine vinegar

2 tablespoons grated
   Parmesan cheese

1 teaspoon dried Italian seasoning

1 teaspoon dried basil leaves

⅛ teaspoon celery salt

⅛ teaspoon freshly ground
   black pepper

In a small jar with a tight-fitting lid, combine the olive oil, vinegar, Parmesan cheese, Italian seasoning, basil, celery salt, and pepper and shake to combine. Refrigerate, covered, up to 1 week.

Ingredient Tip: Other dried herbs can be added to this dressing, including oregano, dill weed, onion powder, and garlic powder.

Per Serving (1 tablespoon) Calories: 94; Total fat: 10g; Saturated fat: 2g; Sodium: 27mg; Phosphorus: 6mg; Potassium: 6mg; Carbohydrates: 1g; Fiber: 0g; Protein: 0g; Sugar: 0g

Creamy Tzatziki Salad Dressing

DIABETES-FRIENDLY, GLUTEN-FREE, HIGH FIBER, LOW PROTEIN, VEGETARIAN

Makes 1 cup / Prep Time: 10 minutes

Tzatziki, pronounced "tsah-SEE-key," is a Greek dressing traditionally made of plain yogurt, chopped cucumber, lemon juice, olive oil and spices. The finished product is cool, creamy, and refreshing. Try it as a dressing in a salad or wrap, or use it as a dip with your favorite raw vegetables. This dressing is incredibly low in sodium, making it a great choice for people with CKD.

1 small cucumber, peeled and grated (about ¾ cup)

⅔ cup plain whole-milk Greek yogurt

2 tablespoons extra-virgin olive oil

1 tablespoon freshly squeezed lemon juice

1 tablespoon chopped fresh mint

1 garlic clove, minced

Pinch salt

In a small bowl, whisk the cucumber, yogurt, olive oil, lemon juice, mint, garlic, and salt until smooth. Store in an airtight container in the refrigerator for up to 1 week.

Ingredient Tip: For a different flavor, try substituting fresh dill weed for the fresh mint.

Per Serving (¼ cup) Calories: 81; Total fat: 8g; Saturated fat: 2g; Sodium: 50mg; Phosphorus: 27mg; Potassium: 94mg; Carbohydrates: 3g; Fiber: 0g; Protein: 1g; Sugar: 2g

Easy Pesto

DIABETES-FRIENDLY, GLUTEN-FREE, LOW PROTEIN, VEGETARIAN

Makes 1 cup / Prep Time: 15 minutes

Pesto is a flavorful Italian no-cook sauce that is made from fresh basil, garlic, and olive oil. You must use fresh basil in this recipe; dried just won't do. It's readily available in grocery stores even during the winter months. The classic way to use pesto is as a sauce for pasta, but you can also use it instead of tomato sauce on a pizza or as a zesty spread on a sandwich.

2 cups fresh basil leaves

3 tablespoons grated
Parmesan cheese

3 tablespoons pine nuts

3 tablespoons extra-virgin olive oil,
plus more for drizzling

2 tablespoons water

1 tablespoon freshly squeezed
lemon juice

2 garlic cloves, sliced

1. In a blender or food processor, combine the basil, Parmesan cheese, pine nuts, olive oil, water, lemon juice, and garlic and blend until the mixture is almost smooth. You can also use a mortar and pestle to grind all the ingredients together.

2. Place the pesto in a small bowl and drizzle more olive oil on top to prevent browning. Store in an airtight container in the refrigerator for up to 3 days.

Make It Easy: You can freeze this pesto to use in recipes. Just spoon the pesto into plastic ice cube trays and freeze up to 3 months. To use, thaw the pesto cubes in the fridge before you add it to the recipes. Or just drop a cube into a pasta sauce or soup and let it cook.

Per Serving (2 tablespoons) Calories: 39; Total fat: 4g; Saturated fat: 1g; Sodium: 23mg; Phosphorus: 11mg; Potassium: 29mg; Carbohydrates: 1g; Fiber: 0g; Protein: 1g; Sugar: 0g

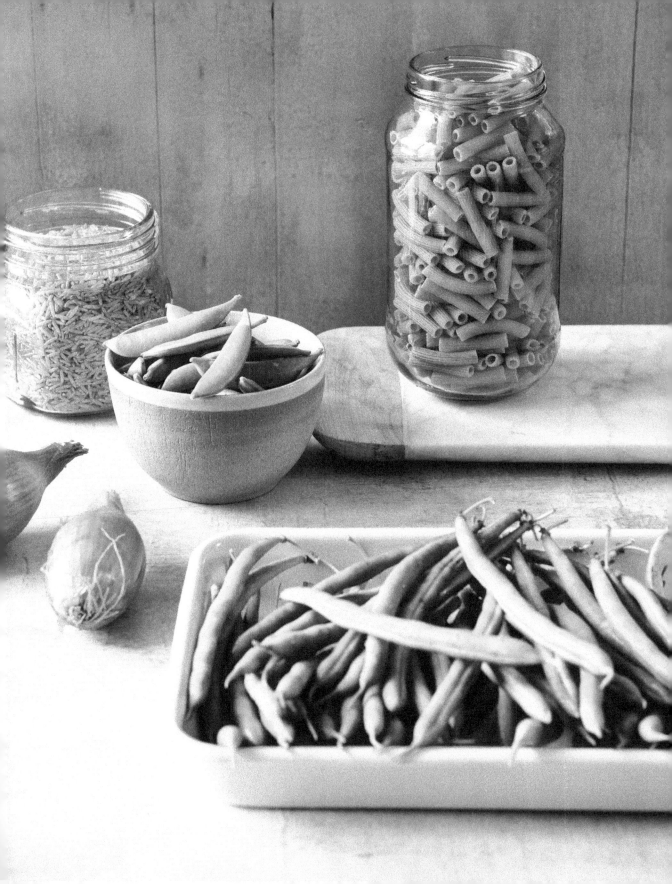

FOOD LISTS FOR THE RENAL DIET

POTASSIUM

HIGHER-POTASSIUM LEGUMES*

Greater than 300 mg per cooked ½ cup serving

Pinto beans	Kidney beans
Lentils	Black beans

LOWER-POTASSIUM LEGUMES

Less than 300 mg per serving listed

¼ cup chopped peanuts	½ cup chickpeas	2 tablespoons
4 oz tofu		peanut butter

HIGHER-POTASSIUM NUTS

Greater than 200 mg per ¼ cup serving

Pistachios (shelled)	Cashews	Almonds
Brazil nuts	Pine nuts	

LOWER-POTASSIUM NUTS

Less than 200 mg per ¼ cup serving

Pecans	Walnuts	Macadamia nuts

HIGHER-POTASSIUM SEAFOOD

Greater than 300 mg per cooked 3 oz serving, unless otherwise specified

Salmon	Atlantic mackerel	4 raw oysters
Trout	Tilapia	
Sardines	4 clams	

LOWER-POTASSIUM SEAFOOD

Less than 300 mg per cooked 3 oz serving (unless otherwise specified)

Cod	Shrimp	Sole
Sea bass	Crab	Flounder
Scallops	Lobster	

*These higher-potassium legumes can fit into a low-potassium diet as long as you stick to the serving size and avoid combining with higher-potassium vegetables, grains and/or meat/poultry/fish.

HIGHER-POTASSIUM MEAT, POULTRY, AND EGGS

Greater than 300 mg per cooked 3 oz serving (unless otherwise specified)

Pork chop	Pork tenderloin	Steak

LOWER-POTASSIUM MEAT, POULTRY, AND EGGS

Less than 300 mg per cooked 3 oz serving (unless otherwise specified)

Veal	Turkey breast	3 egg whites
Lamb	Chicken breast	2 eggs
Hamburger	Chicken thigh	

HIGHER-POTASSIUM DAIRY AND DAIRY ALTERNATIVE FOODS

Greater than 300 mg per serving specified

1 cup evaporated milk	5-ounce container of	1 cup whole milk
1 cup low-fat milk	low-fat, plain yogurt	1 cup soy milk

LOWER-POTASSIUM DAIRY AND DAIRY ALTERNATIVE FOODS

Less than 300 mg per serving specified

5-ounce container of low-fat, plain Greek yogurt	5-ounce container of whole-milk, Greek yogurt	5-ounce cottage cheese
5-ounce container of whole-milk, plain yogurt	5-ounce almond-milk-based plain yogurt	½ cup chocolate ice cream
1 cup rice milk, unenriched		1 cup almond milk
		½ cup vanilla ice cream
		1 oz cheese (most types)

HIGHER-POTASSIUM GRAINS AND STARCHES (MG) **

Greater than 200 mg per cooked 1 cup serving (unless otherwise specified)

1 boiled skinless medium white potato*	1 boiled skinless medium sweet potato*	Quinoa

LOWER-POTASSIUM GRAINS AND STARCHES (MG)

Less than 200 mg per cooked 1 cup serving (unless otherwise specified)

Steel-cut oats	Wild rice	Polenta
2 medium slices whole-wheat bread	Pearled barley	2 medium slices rye bread
Bulgur	Old-fashioned oats	Couscous
Peas	1 whole-wheat English muffin	Spaghetti
Brown rice	Whole-wheat spaghetti	White rice

**High-potassium root vegetables, such as potatoes, can be double-boiled to reduce their potassium content. Simply peel, slice and dice your potatoes and place in boiling water for 15 minutes. Drain, add new fresh water, and cook until done.

HIGHER-POTASSIUM FRUITS (MG)

More than 200 mg per ½ cup fresh, canned, or 1 small fruit (unless otherwise specified)

Avocado

Banana

Dried fruit: raisins, dates, figs, apricots, bananas, peaches, pears, or prunes (¼ cup)

Honeydew

Kiwi

Nectarine

Orange

Papaya

Peach

Plantain

Pomegranate

LOWER-POTASSIUM FRUITS (MG)

Less than 200 mg per ½ cup fresh, canned, or 1 small fruit (unless otherwise specified)

Apple

Applesauce

Apricot, fresh

Berries

Cherries

Clementine

Dried apples, blueberries, cherries, or cranberries (¼ cup)

Fruit cup: any fruit, fruit cocktail

Grapes

Lemon or lime

Pear

Pineapple

Plum

Tangerine or mandarin orange

Watermelon (1 cup)

HIGHER-POTASSIUM VEGETABLES (MG)

More than 200 mg per 1 cup leafy greens or ½ cup fresh, cooked or canned vegetables (unless otherwise specified)

Acorn squash

Artichoke

Beet greens

Brussels sprouts

Butternut squash

Chard (cooked)

Chinese cabbage (cooked)

Corn (1 ear)

Edamame

Hubbard squash

Kohlrabi

Lentils

Parsnips

Potatoes

Pumpkins

Rutabaga

Spinach (cooked)

Tomato

Tomato sauce, tomato paste, tomato juice

Yams

Zucchini

Vegetable juice

Less than 200 mg per 1 cup leafy greens or ½ cup
Fresh, cooked, or canned vegetables (unless otherwise specified)

Alfalfa sprouts

Asparagus

Bamboo shoots (canned)

Bean sprouts

Beets (canned)

Broccoli

Cabbage

Carrots

Cauliflower

Celery

Cucumber

Eggplant

Green or wax beans

Greens: collard, mustard,
   or turnip

Jicama/yambean

Kale

Lettuce: all types

Mushrooms (raw
   or canned)

Okra

Onion or leek

Peas: green, sugar snap,
   or snow peas

Peppers: green, red,
   or yellow

Radish

Rhubarb

Spinach (raw)

Spaghetti squash

Cherry tomatoes

Turnip

Yellow summer squash

Water chestnuts (canned)

PROTEIN

Protein-rich foods include meat, poultry, fish, eggs, milk, cheese, legumes, nuts, and grains. Fruits and vegetables contain very low amounts of protein and therefore are not included.

Per ½ cup serving cooked, unless otherwise specified

Soybeans 16

4 oz silken tofu, not
   silken 15

4 oz silken tofu 10

Lentils 9

¼ cup peanuts 9

Pinto beans 8

Kidney beans 8

Black beans 8

Chickpeas 7

2 tablespoons peanut
   butter 7

Per ¼ cup serving, unless otherwise specified

Almonds 7

Cashews 6

Pistachios 6

Walnuts 5

Brazil nuts 5

Pine nuts 4

Pecans 3

Macadamia nuts 2

PROTEIN IN GRAINS AND STARCHES (G)

Per 1 cup serving cooked, unless otherwise specified

2 medium slices
  whole-wheat bread 9

Quinoa 8

Peas 8

Whole-wheat or regular
  spaghetti 8

Steel-cut oats 7

Wild rice 7

Old-fashioned oats 6

Brown rice 6

Bulgur 6

Couscous 6

Whole-wheat English
  muffin 6

2 medium slices
  rye bread 5

Pearled barley 5

Polenta/grits 4

White rice 4

PROTEIN IN SEAFOOD (G)

Per 3 oz serving cooked, unless otherwise specified

Sardines 22

Salmon 22

Tilapia 22

Shrimp 20

Atlantic mackerel 20

Trout 20

Sea bass 20

Scallops 18

Cod 17

4 raw oysters 17

Lobster 16

Crab 15

Sole 13

Flounder 13

4 clams 12

PROTEIN IN MEAT, POULTRY, AND EGGS (G)

Per 3 oz serving cooked, unless otherwise specified

Turkey breast 26

Chicken breast 26

Pork chop 25

Steak 25

Chicken thigh 24

Pork tenderloin 24

Lamb 24

Hamburger 22

Veal 21

2 eggs 13

3 egg whites 11

PROTEIN IN DAIRY AND DAIRY-ALTERNATIVE FOODS (G)

Per 1 cup serving, unless otherwise specified

1 cup evaporated milk 17

5 oz low-fat cottage
  cheese 15

5 oz container of low-fat,
  plain Greek yogurt 15

5 oz container of
  whole-milk, Greek
  yogurt 13

1 oz cheese (most
  types) 6-8

1 cup low-fat milk 8

1 cup whole milk 8

1 cup soy milk 8

5 oz container of low-fat,
  plain yogurt 7

5 oz almond milk-based
  plain yogurt 6

5 oz container of
  whole-milk, plain
  yogurt 5

½ cup ice cream 3

1 cup rice milk,
  unenriched 2

1 cup almond milk 1

SODIUM

Check food labels for actual sodium content per serving

Table salt

Most canned foods (unless specified no salt added or low-sodium)

Bread

Seasoning salt

Ham

Sauerkraut

Soy sauce

Sausage

Fast foods

Teriyaki sauce

Microwave meals

Salad dressings

Garlic salt

Potato chips

Hot dogs

Onion salt

Salted crackers

Cold cuts, deli meat

Spam

Buttermilk

Corned beef

Vegetable juices

Canned ravioli

Frozen prepared foods

Barbecue sauce

Bouillon cubes

Bacon

Smoked fish

Baking mixes (pancakes, desserts)

Steak sauce

Monosodium glutamate (MSG)

Ketchup

High-sodium cereals

Check food labels for actual sodium content per serving

Fresh garlic

Low-sodium salad dressings

Canned food with no added salt

Fresh onion

Allspice

Low-sodium seasoning blends

Black pepper

Ginger

Fresh fish

Lemon juice

Rosemary

Eggs

Vinegar, regular or flavored

Thyme

Dry mustard

Nuts, unsalted

Unsalted popcorn

Sage

Pretzels, unsalted

Homemade or no salt added broth

Tarragon

Crackers, unsalted

Lower sodium breads and cereals (check label)

Dill

PHOSPHORUS

Phosphorus is found in protein-rich foods. Fruits and vegetables contain very low amounts of phosphorus and therefore are not included. Tables include total phosphorus and phosphorus adjusted for estimated bioavailability in descending order.

Plant Sources of Phosphorus: Low Bioavailability

*Adjusted phosphorus is based on the estimated 50% bioavailability of phosphorus in plant sources.

PHOSPHORUS IN LEGUMES (MG)

Per ½ cup serving cooked, unless otherwise specified

FOOD	PHOSPHORUS	ADJUSTED PHOSPHORUS*
Soybeans	211	106
Lentils	178	89
Chickpeas	138	69
¼ cup peanuts	137	69
Pinto beans	126	63
Kidney beans	122	61
4 oz tofu, not silken	122	61
Black beans	120	60
2 tablespoons peanut butter	108	54
4 oz silken tofu	102	51

PHOSPHORUS IN NUTS (MG)

Per ¼ cup serving

FOOD	PHOSPHORUS	ADJUSTED PHOSPHORUS*
Brazil nuts	241	121
Pine nuts	194	97
Cashews	191	96
Almonds	156	78
Pistachios	151	76
Walnuts	101	51
Pecans	76	38
Macadamia nuts	63	32

FOOD	PHOSPHORUS	ADJUSTED PHOSPHORUS*
1 cup cooked quinoa	281	141
1 cup cooked steel-cut oats	219	110
1 cup cooked brown rice	208	104
1 cup cooked whole-wheat spaghetti	178	89
1 cup cooked old-fashioned oats	172	86
1 cup cooked wild rice	135	68
1 cup cooked bulgur	134	67
1 cup cooked pearled barley	121	61
1 cup cooked couscous	80	40
1 cup cooked polenta/grits	53	27

ANIMAL SOURCES OF PHOSPHORUS: MEDIUM BIOAVAILABILITY

*Adjusted phosphorus is based on the estimated 70-percent bioavailability of phosphorus in animal sources.

PHOSPHORUS IN SEAFOOD (MG)

Per 3 oz serving cooked, unless otherwise specified

FOOD	PHOSPHORUS	ADJUSTED PHOSPHORUS*
Scallops	362	253
4 raw oysters	294	206
Sardines	272	190
Sole	263	184
Flounder	262	183
Atlantic mackerel	236	165
Trout	230	161
Salmon	218	153
Sea bass	211	148
Shrimp	202	141
Crab	199	139
Tilapia	174	122
4 clams	164	115
Lobster	157	81
Light tuna	139	97
Cod	117	82

Phosphorus Cooking Tip: Research shows that preparing meats by boiling them in liquid can reduce the phosphorus content by 10 to 50 percent. This works best when the meat is sliced before cooking. Because the phosphorus is leached into the liquid, you'll need to discard the cooking liquid before serving.

Per 3 oz serving cooked, unless otherwise specified

FOOD	PHOSPHORUS	ADJUSTED PHOSPHORUS*
Pork tenderloin	248	174
Steak	230	161
Turkey breast	196	137
Veal	190	133
Pork chop	189	132
Chicken breast	184	129
Chicken thigh	180	126
Lamb	173	121
Hamburger	158	111
2 eggs	172	120
Hamburger	158	111
3 egg whites	15	11

PHOSPHORUS IN DAIRY FOODS (G)

Per serving size listed

FOOD	PHOSPHORUS	ADJUSTED PHOSPHORUS*
1 cup evaporated milk	460	322
1 cup low-fat milk	225	158
5 oz low-fat cottage cheese	213	149
1 cup whole milk	205	144
5 oz container of low-fat, plain yogurt	204	143
5 oz container of whole-milk, Greek yogurt	191	134
5 oz container of low-fat, plain Greek yogurt	141	99
5 oz container of whole-milk, plain yogurt	135	95
1 oz cheese (most types)	130–180	91–126
1 oz Feta cheese	96	67
1 oz Goat cheese	73	51
½ cup ice cream	69	48
1 oz Brie cheese	53	37

PROCESSED SOURCES OF PHOSPHORUS: HIGH BIOAVAILABILITY (80–100%)

The food industry is not required to provide the phosphorus content of processed foods. Foods with phosphorus additives represent the most bioavailable form of phosphorus in the diet. The following foods frequently contain phosphorus additives. Always check the ingredients of foods to be sure.

Fast food ("fast-fresh" food may be okay)

Bottled drinks such as soda, flavored waters, and juices

Certain brands of non-dairy creamers or half-and-half

Certain brands of non-dairy milks

Processed meats (includes all cold cuts as well as breakfast meats such as sausage, bacon and turkey bacon)

Frozen prepared meals

Many canned foods

Processed sweet and savory snack foods (cakes, cookies, and cheese-based snacks)

HIGH-FIBER CARBOHYDRATES

Fiber is found in vegetables, fruits, whole grains, nuts, and legumes.

HIGH-FIBER LEGUMES (G)

Per ½ cup serving cooked, unless otherwise specified

Pinto beans 8

Black beans 8

Kidney beans 6

Lentils 6

Chickpeas 5

HIGH-FIBER NUTS (G)

Per ¼ cup serving

Almonds 4

Brazil nuts 3

Pecans 3

Macadamia nuts 3

Pistachios 3

Per 1 cup cooked, unless otherwise specified

Old-fashioned oats 8

Peas 7

Whole-wheat spaghetti 6

Bulgur 6

Steel-cut oats 5

Quinoa 5

1 medium sweet potato 4

1 medium white potato 4

2 medium slices
whole-wheat bread 4

Whole-wheat English
muffin 4

Brown rice 3

2 medium slices
rye bread 3

Per ½ cup fresh, canned, or 1 small fruit unless otherwise specified

Pear 6

Apple 4

Blackberries 4

Raspberries 4

Blueberries 2

Strawberries 2

¼ avocado 2

Mandarin orange 2

Per ½ cup cooked, unless otherwise specified

Collard greens 4

Brussels sprouts 3

Broccoli 3

Asparagus 2

Carrots 2

Green beans 2

Mushrooms 2

1 cup raw baby spinach 1

Cauliflower 1

HEART-HEALTHY FATS

Olive oil

Avocado oil

Sesame oil

Flaxseed oil (keep
refrigerated and do
not heat)

Hemp oil (keep
refrigerated and avoid
high heat)

Sesame oil (keep
refrigerated and avoid
high heat)

Walnut oil (keep
refrigerated and avoid
high heat)

Salmon

Atlantic mackerel (avoid
king mackerel due to
mercury content)

Rainbow trout

Sardines

NUTS/NUT BUTTERS AND SEEDS

Peanuts and peanut butter

Almonds and
    almond butter

Walnuts

Cashews

Brazil nuts

Pine nuts

Pecans

Macadamia nuts

Pistachios

Sunflower seeds

Flaxseed

Chia seeds

MISCELLANEOUS

Avocado

Low-sodium olives

Measurement Conversions

	US STANDARD	US STANDARD (OUNCES)	METRIC (APPROXIMATE)
VOLUME EQUIVALENTS (LIQUID)	2 tablespoons	1 fl. oz.	30 mL
	¼ cup	2 fl. oz.	60 mL
	½ cup	4 fl. oz.	120 mL
	1 cup	8 fl. oz.	240 mL
	1½ cups	12 fl. oz.	355 mL
	2 cups or 1 pint	16 fl. oz.	475 mL
	4 cups or 1 quart	32 fl. oz.	1 L
	1 gallon	128 fl. oz.	4 L
VOLUME EQUIVALENTS (DRY)	⅛ teaspoon		0.5 mL
	¼ teaspoon		1 mL
	½ teaspoon		2 mL
	¾ teaspoon		4 mL
	1 teaspoon		5 mL
	1 tablespoon		15 mL
	¼ cup		59 mL
	⅓ cup		79 mL
	½ cup		118 mL
	⅔ cup		156 mL
	¾ cup		177 mL
	1 cup		235 mL
	2 cups or 1 pint		475 mL
	3 cups		700 mL
	4 cups or 1 quart		1 L
	½ gallon		2 L
	1 gallon		4 L
WEIGHT EQUIVALENTS	½ ounce		15 g
	1 ounce		30 g
	2 ounces		60 g
	4 ounces		115 g
	8 ounces		225 g
	12 ounces		340 g
	16 ounces or 1 pound		455 g

	FAHRENHEIT (F)	CELSIUS (C) (APPROXIMATE)
OVEN TEMPERATURES	250°F	120°C
	300°F	150°C
	325°F	180°C
	375°F	190°C
	400°F	200°C
	425°F	220°C
	450°F	230°C

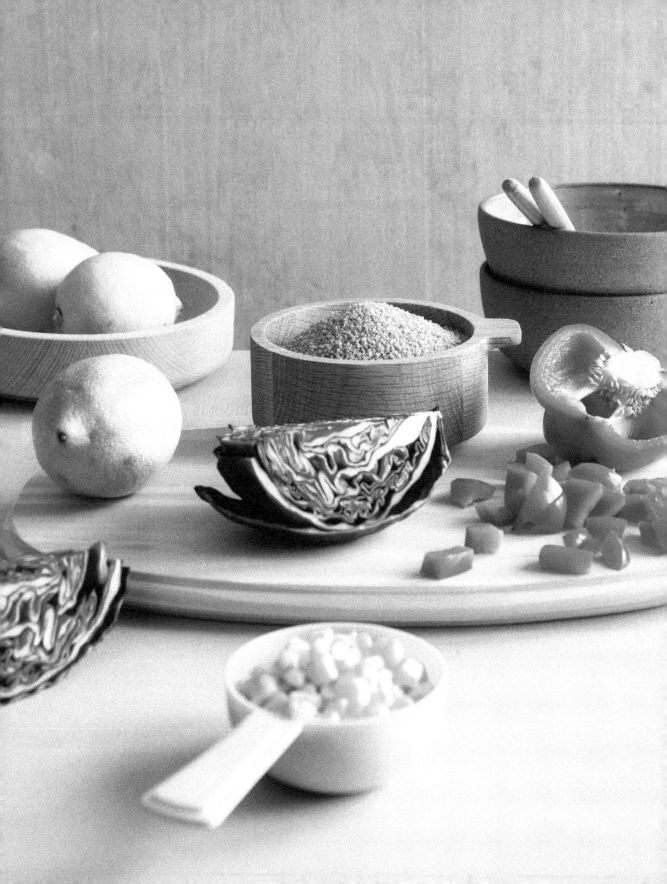

Index

Acknowledgments

Thank you to Linda Larsen for your hard work and dedication on the project. Your collaboration helped this book shine and means tasty recipes for everyone!

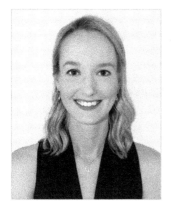

Aisling Whelan is a registered dietitian who uses a whole-person, whole-food-based approach to help clients reclaim their health and improve their quality of life. She completed her didactic program in dietetics at Simmons University in Boston and obtained a master's degree in clinical nutrition from New York University. Aisling has extensive experience working with the chronic kidney disease population. Her first introduction to renal nutrition began when she worked as a dietitian in a hemodialysis facility. In this role, Aisling was surprised to learn that most of her patients had never met with a dietitian prior to starting dialysis. It was this discovery that inspired Aisling to start her own private practice specializing in nutrition therapy for pre-dialysis CKD patients. Aisling is passionate about empowering her patients to implement realistic and sustainable changes aimed at slowing down the progression of their kidney disease. In addition to specializing in kidney disease, Aisling also has expertise in treating other conditions such as diabetes, obesity, hypertension, and women's health issues. Aisling lives with her husband and son in New York City.

CPSIA information can be obtained
at www.ICGtesting.com
Printed in the USA
JSHW051957060921
18502JS00003B/43